More Reviews for The Sun, The Rain and The Insulin.

"What a rewarding book for anyone who knows a child or adult with diabetes. I laughed and I cried with the characters. Teachers, parents, relatives, friends, and others will gain useful information while they enjoy a delightful story."
Sue Owens, former nurse and teacher

"Dr. MacCracken's book fills a vacant niche on my library shelf: that of a personal account of families coping with diabetes. **This book should be in all libraries with consumer health clientele.**"

Sue Jagels, Library Director, Parrot Health Sciences Library

"Diabetes nearly took my life in the Spring of 1995. At the age of 28, I've had it for less than a year and am obviously still learning. This book took me into the lives of people just like me and answered many critical questions -- both medical and social. It is perhaps the most realistic, emotional, and understandable book on the subject I've yet to read. And because of it, I'm healthier, happier, and truly grateful."
Greg Hoel, assistant editor and a "real-live diabetic"

"Every day I share with my patients their experience of chronic disease. I never fully realized the range of feelings illness engenders. It took reading about them in others to recognize them in myself. And then it felt possible to find a place to put them."

Elizabeth Weiss, M.D., mother of child with recently diagnosed diabetes

"Dr. MacCracken's book gives clear, concrete information with examples of how family-centered care can work in practice. I gained an increased understanding and awareness of the multiple issues and stressors that such families deal with."

Susan Knowlton, LCSW, Pediatric Social Worker

The Sun, The Rain, and The Insulin

Growing Up With Diabetes

Joan MacCracken, M.D.

Tiffin Press of Maine

THE SUN, THE RAIN, AND THE INSULIN
Growing Up With Diabetes.

Copyright © 1996 by Joan MacCracken, M.D.

Published by: *TIFFIN PRESS OF MAINE*, Orono, Maine 04473

Editor: Donna Hoel, Minnetonka, Minnesota

Assistant Editor: Greg Hoel, Hopkins, Minnesota

Cover Drawing of Hersey Retreat by: Anne Kilham,
                                                 Rockport, Maine

Design Consultant: Brad Finch, Northeast Reprographics,
                                                 Bangor, Maine

Note to the reader: This book recounts the essence of my experience and in that sense is a true story. The camp, staff, and location are real. However, the book is not intended as a literal account, and all names and details of the campers and counselors are fictitious and are not to be taken as a portrayal of any living person.

Library of Congress Catalog Card Number: 96-90047

Publisher's Cataloging-in-Publication Data
        MacCracken, Joan, M.D.(1945 -   )
        The Sun, The Rain, and The Insulin
        Growing Up with Diabetes
                1. Diabetes—Popular works   2. Children—Diseases
        ISBN 0-9646018-5-0

Printed by: **McNaughton & Gunn, Inc., Saline, Michigan**
on 50% recycled fiber paper in the United States of America.

To all the families with diabetes
who have taught me so much

and

To my father and my mother

■■■■■■■■■■■■■■■■■
Acknowledgments

Along the path to completion of this project, I received much encouragement and support from both old and new friends. Without it, the journey would have been rougher and I might have run out of energy and confidence to persevere.

Role models in endocrinology and pediatric diabetology inspired me to pursue my clinical endocrine career. Thanks to Dr. Olof Pearson, Dr. Ruth Owens, and Dr. Dorothy Becker.

In the very beginning my step-mother, Mary MacCracken, told me to write down my memorable experiences. I finally took her advice. Thanks to her and so many friends who have read and commented on my manuscript and who bolstered me as the larger publishing companies politely rejected my project. Thank you Jeem Trowbridge, Susan Jagels, Juan Bayer, Claire McKnight, Betsy Weiss, Chris Happel, Joyceann Yaccarino, Mike Stenger, Don and Ann Pilcher, Susan Knowlton, Jan Donaldson, Jennifer Pixley, Wendy Satin-Rapaport, Sue Owens, Sandy Hutchins, Stu Brink, and Anne Woodbury.

Of course, without the special team at camp, it never would be the fun, enjoyable experience we all look forward to each year. A tremendous thanks to Cindy Hale, Laurie Ward, Tim Rogers, Heather Leclerc, and especially to Pat Stenger, who has been my partner in all our family diabetes projects. She is a treasure for diabetes education and advocacy and for me. Thanks, Pat, for being such a long-standing, invaluable friend.

From my long first draft to the rewritten manuscript to his gracious foreword, Dr. Allan Drash has been one of my major supporters. I wish him well on his retirement from Children's Hospital of Pittsburgh this year.

Anne Kilham captured the peacefulness and beauty of our Maine coast with her cover drawing. I appreciate her artistry and thank her for taking a phone call from a total stranger. Brad Finch, my design consultant, gave me two words of advice, "Don't panic!" Thanks.

Relentless in her enthusiasm and support, Donna Hoel, formerly of Chronimed, has fought for my cause. She believed in my book even before her own son Greg came down with diabetes. I owe her much for her confidence and am very proud and lucky to have her as my editor.

And when the trail had led to an impasse and I was in a stall, Lynda Clyve, whom I have known for 19 years in Bangor, gave me a final lift. Thanks for your generous financial and emotional support.

Finally, to all my family, particularly my brother, Michael, and my mother, who showed me the way to self-publishing and to my husband Bob Holmberg and my children Tim and Molly, who carried on with the household duties as I drifted off mentally running through those author/publisher to-do lists, thanks! At last, it's a reality.

Joan MacCracken, M.D.

Table of Contents

Foreword

Diabetes mellitus is one of the most common serious chronic diseases of childhood. It has extraordinary impact on our health care system, with total diabetes health care expenses (for all age groups) accounting for approximately 15 percent of all health care costs in the United States.

Approximately 250,000 children and adolescents in the U.S. have insulin-dependent diabetes. The prevalence rate is about 3 cases per 1,000, with an incidence or attack rate of approximately 15 new cases per 100,000 per year. There is evidence that these numbers are growing.

Many Americans are aware of the dreaded complications of diabetes mellitus, including blindness, renal failure, and nerve and vascular damage. The Diabetes Control and Complications Trial (DCCT), which recently ended after nine years of research, clearly showed that the serious complications of this disease can be reduced or minimized by aggressive, intensive diabetes management.

All of us involved in diabetes care around the world have taken the DCCT results seriously and are attempting to improve our management package to ensure a better life for our patients. It is a major challenge that involves the patient as the central participant in the therapeutic team. However, the extended team must also involve parents, siblings, physicians, nurse educators, dietitians, behavioral scientists, and many individuals in the local community, such as teachers and coaches.

Much less well appreciated than the vascular complications of diabetes are the emotional consequences that so commonly accompany this disorder. Living with diabetes day-by-day is a heavy burden. It is particularly difficult for the adolescent in the midst of fighting for independence of parents, teachers, and other authoritative individuals and institutions.

In long-term prospective studies carried out in our clinic at the Children's Hospital of Pittsburgh, we find that about 50 percent of children with insulin-dependent diabetes have at least one serious psychiatric episode as they go through adolescence and become established as young adults. In most cases this is a major depressive disease. In such individuals, recurrent depression is likely. In children who do not become depressed but have other emotional problems, a variety of behaviors may be seen, such as aggressive antisocial behavior, withdrawal, school failure and dropout, alcoholism, and drug abuse.

The best preventive approach to the behavioral disabilities so commonly seen in teenagers with diabetes mellitus is a strong, supportive family who can gain strength and direction from a team of professionals who are sensitive to behavioral issues and act on them appropriately when identified.

Dr. Joan MacCracken has written an important book. *The Sun, The Rain, and the Insulin: Growing Up With Diabetes* is unique in the diabetes literature. The setting is a diabetes family camp in Maine. Through a series of vignettes, Dr. MacCracken provides examples of potential family concerns, including compliance issues, acting-out behaviors, immaturity, and rejection of the disease by both patients and parents. Much more importantly, we are taken through the steps of resolution in a real-life arena. In many cases, problems are worked out. But, as is always the case, there are also some failures.

This book can serve as a detailed road map—a "how-you-do-it" in the day-to-day management of diabetes. It can provide extraordinarily important insights for the older patients and certainly for parents of children with diabetes. It also will be a valuable tool for diabetes professionals and others who interact with children with diabetes, including teachers and coaches.

I heartily endorse this book, knowing that it can provide comfort, education, and direction for its readers.

Allen L. Drash, M.D.
Children's Hospital of Pittsburgh

Preface

In the next decade or two, diabetes care will be very different. In fact, the disease itself may even be preventable. But for now, there are thousands of families facing the daily task of managing diabetes. And that's not easy.

The diagnosis brings the startling realization that your child's life will be dramatically altered, and even your family's life will never be the same. In time the routine will become easier. But the haunting questions of why and how, the frustrating times of juggling the multiple components that affect blood sugar, and the worry of an uncertain future will linger.

Facing these concerns alone is not necessary. Diabetes centers throughout the country are working to improve the lives of these children and adults with diabetes.

At Eastern Maine Medical Center, we have successfully included the families in the educational process. I feel our greatest contribution has been the creation of Camp Kee-To-Kin, a camp for families with diabetes. Here parents, children, grandparents, and significant others come together and share their deepest concerns. They cry and they laugh. With education, encouragement, and mutual support the families gain hope. I am very privileged to share our special story of families learning to deal with the challenges of diabetes.

Joan MacCracken, M.D.
Bangor, Maine

Introduction

It all happens right here—a rainbow of emotions, a microcosm of personalities, an incredible mix of lifestyles. Families bring their mental suitcases filled with fears and frustrations, anxieties and angers, questions and guarded anticipation of help. Total strangers, captive for a week, are drawn together by a common thread, diabetes.

I have no illusions that it's easier now, even after nine successful years. Others think our diabetes team is on vacation, away from the hospital for a week with such great surroundings and, usually, good weather. We know we work. But we also know it's worth it.

When Pat, our diabetes nurse educator, and I first thought about the idea of a diabetes family camp, it was just a dream. We had both attended church-sponsored family camps that were such fun—several families together for a week with delicious meals provided. What a break for the mothers. We adults relaxed and put our work responsibilities on the shelf or our busy routines on hold. And the location, Hersey Retreat, provided such an extraordinary environment—the magical sea, the changing tides, the sun's reflection on the water, the colorful sunsets, the smell, the salt air, and the solitude of the Retreat, perched high on the sandy bluff. Time stood still.

Why not bring people here for a week, let them learn more

about diabetes while living and sharing with other families in a fun and beautiful place. Our plan was met with cool, if not totally frigid, responses from several individuals.

One pediatrician told us it would just be a miserable week, with each family bringing their germs and spreading them. By the end of the week everyone would be sick. Really? we shrugged. Another rather blunt, yet honest, father told us the last thing he would want to do with his vacation was spend it with a lot of unknown families. He didn't think this concept would fly.

With this initial less than encouraging response, we proceeded on our own. There was no funding available. Our hospital was not interested in supporting such a wild idea. We talked with parents of children with diabetes, and they were more positive. I took out a savings account. Pat and I started asking, begging for money. We literally passed the hat around at the next diabetes support meeting. We needed funding to sponsor families that could not afford to pay. Our church women's group was willing to sponsor one family.

Fortunately, we were able to rent the Retreat for one week for a very reasonable rate. With more work we were almost ready to begin the more formal arrangements—like setting dates, determining costs, planning programs, advertising camp, and signing up families. But first, we needed one more vital player, a dietitian, well educated in diabetes and crazy enough to want to do this with us. Luckily, we found her right under our noses. Cindy worked as the dietitian for the Maine Diabetes Control Project in Augusta. She was very excited about the idea, and the Project gave her the time off. The fact that she had had diabetes since age 18 was an enormous asset.

We plunged ahead, and on June 25, 1982, the front doors of Hersey Retreat were opened to start the first diabetes family camp, which we called Camp Kee-To-Kin. And now, years later, we're still at it. But this year I want to tell the story.

The Cast of Characters

Camp Kee-To-Kin

Wright Family—Sam, Pearl (grandmother), *Emily (5)

Stone Family—Lydia, *Kevin (11), Cindy (13)

Booth Family—Brent, Marjorie, *Susan (10), Tate (6)

Russell Family—Darryl, Nancy, *Becky (12)

McCabe Family—Mark, Lisa, *Peter (10),

Abigail (8), Lucy (4)

Peterson Family—Lucy, *Jeffrey (7), Kyle (8)

Counselors—Eddy Jelkepski (17),

Ginny Milsom (18)

Staff—Joan MacCracken, M.D., Camp Doctor

Pat Stenger, R.N., Diabetes Nurse Educator

Heather Leclerc, R.D., Dietitian

Tim Rogers, Ph.D., Psychologist

Laurie Ward, Cook

* These children are learning to live with diabetes.

BIRDSEYE VIEW OF He

PENOBSCOT BAY

BEACH

SANDY CLIFFS

SEAL ROCK

GAZEBO

K

ROCKY BEACH

WOODS

VOLLEYBALL

SWINGS

WATERSLIDE

L

ROAD TO BEACH

WOODS

Dri

E

S

N

W

WHITE CABIN

STAFF QUARTERS

SEY RETREAT

LOW TIDE

MUD FLATS

CLAY BANKS

YING FIELD

BIRCHES

SANDBOX

OGE

TIRE SWING

CAMP FIRE

BASEBALL DIAMOND

PATH TO BEACH

RED HOUSE (PRIVATELY OWNED)

LUPINE FIELD.

WOODS

FRENCH HOUSE (OLDEST BUILDING IN WALDO COUNTY)

RSEY RCHT

SANDY POINT, MAINE

Assembling the Players

A red Chevy pickup heads down the driveway. The slow, careful speed indicates strangers are on board. As the truck swings around the loop, we notice two passengers, a woman and a little girl. The driver, a young bearded man, leans out and asks, "Is this Camp Kee-To-Kin?"

"Yep, sure is. You must be Sam," Pat says. "Welcome!"

She glances over at me. Our thoughts at that moment are one. Here we go again. Let's do it!

It astounds me how Pat remembers names so well. I'm always worried that I'll never be able to learn the names of so many new faces, all arriving at once. I try to look over the list, which she provides me, but until I have a face to put with a name, it just doesn't help much.

By 4:30 all six families are here. With our help they locate their rooms and carry their luggage up the broad staircase. The bedrooms vary in size from quite small, just enough for a dresser and twin bed (Ginny, our counselor, gets this room right at the head of the stairs), to very large, with three to four bunk beds and a double bed.

Families enjoy setting up their own arrangements, assigning the upper bunks and protecting the little ones from falls in the night. Some push bunks together, others place mattresses on the floor in case of a tumble. The variety of paraphernalia that campers bring is fascinating. Some look as if they'll be staying for a month.

The Retreat provides sheets and blankets, but many bring sleeping bags, which most kids prefer; it's more like camping out, and you don't have to make them in the morning. Having the entire family sleep all in one room for a week is a change for most. We find this gives each family some needed privacy, and in a new setting the kids are more comfortable. We're certainly more comfortable, too, knowing that the parents are with their kids, still ultimately responsible for their welfare and behavior. Pat and I realize this is a great advantage of family camp.

At 5 o'clock, we ring the bell in the hallway, hoping everyone realizes we are trying to call a meeting. With a few messengers sent upstairs, the group slowly assembles in the meeting room. Everyone is here but Heather, our dietitian. She replaced our first dietitian, Cindy, about four years ago, but still gets lost finding camp. She'll be here soon, I'm sure.

"Welcome to all of you. If you haven't met me yet, I'm Pat Stenger, and to my right here is Dr. MacCracken. Our two counselors this year are Ginny and Eddy." Eddy bows. "Heather, our dietitian, should be arriving shortly. We're delighted that you were all able to find the Retreat without too much difficulty."

"Daddy, got lost three times!" says a small little boy, who sits on his mother's lap.

"Well, then, a special welcome to you who almost got lost." Everyone smiles.

"We'll eat at 5:30 in the French House, that white building on the other side of the red house. And after supper, around 7 o'clock, we'll meet here to learn more about the Retreat, our schedule, and each other. For those of you who do blood testing before supper and take insulin, this would be a good time to do that."

Campers start to move. "We'll ring the bell when they're ready for us in the French House. Check the bulletin board for the list of dishwashers for breakfast and supper. Tonight the job goes to . . ." Pat looks down at her paper, "Lisa, Brent, and Abigail." Everyone leaves the room except the almost lost little boy, who starts pounding on the old piano keys.

Heather pulls her gray Subaru in the driveway as the supper bell rings. We all walk over to dinner and fill the two rather small rooms. As usual at the first meal, most of the family members sit with each other at one of the four rectangular tables. As the week proceeds, this will change. Parents will allow their kids to sit in the other room out of their sight. Kids will want to sit with their newly made friends, and the adults will enjoy sharing conversations, perhaps slowly savoring their second cup of coffee. But, tonight there is an understandable shyness, reticence, and hush. We're still strangers.

At supper I sit with two very different families. To my right is a family from Philadelphia, who took two days to drive up. Brent, a math professor, tells me he and his wife, Marjorie, summered as teenagers in Blue Hill. They've been eager to return to Maine to show their two younger children the area. Their two older children have summer jobs in Maine. The professor, tall, dark, and rather lanky, wears a faded Lacoste knit shirt and madras bermuda shorts.

"Susan's our diabetic," says Brent. His daughter looks at me with a half-smile, half-glare. I understand. She obviously doesn't like being referred to as *our diabetic.* "And Tate has just come along for the ride. Right, Tater?"

"Daddy, you know I get carsick. I hate the ride. But I think I'll like it here!" With a typical six-year-old's toothless grin, he smiles.

Marjorie, a slightly heavy version of Meryl Streep, nudges her son, Tate, suggesting that he better eat his dinner. His meatloaf, loaded with ketchup, is hardly touched. Tate slowly obeys.

On my left are three other campers. The overweight boy of 10 or 11 requests more bread. He piles on the margarine and rapidly consumes the slice. Across the table from him is a teenage girl whose eyes are fixed on the table. Her long, dark scraggly hair covers most of her face. Her old navy blue "Laura B Monhegan Boat" sweatshirt catches my eye.

"Have you been to Monhegan?" I ask, trying to catch her attention. She looks up as if to speak, but the very large woman at the head of the table answers instead.

"Naw, we just get the leftovers from the thrift shop in Port Clyde. Not too bad a place actually . . . . Kevin, don't take any more bread. You've had enough." She grabs his hand as he reaches for another piece.

"So, Kevin, you live in Port Clyde?"

"Yeah, but I wish I lived somewhere else. It's . . . ."

"Oh, Kev, you always say that," says the teenage girl, presumably his sister.

"Cindy, why don't you just keep out of this," fires Kevin.

"Cindy, don't interrupt your brother." Her mother glares at her. Cindy resumes her head-down position. I decide to change the subject and ask Kevin's mother to please pass the coffee.

The French House has gone through several renovations but still has the atmosphere of an old home. The ceilings are low and the wide pine board floors are original. Small paned windows allow views of the Penobscot River and open fields filled with purple and pink lupine.

Evenings are at their longest now, so the sun is still well above the hillside as the dishwashers start their job.

At 7 o'clock, the campers head for the meeting room. Two boys swing on the large tire outside. Tate, the little boy who gets carsick, rides his bike around the porch. What a great way to burn off energy; just ride around and around. One girl sits on the steps with her Walkman radio. She taps her foot as she flips the pages of a magazine. The parents of these children round them up, and soon everyone is seated in a big circle in the meeting room. Two of the smallest children sit on their mothers' laps.

Pat starts, "I hope you all had a good supper and are beginning to learn your way around. Before our get-acquainted game, I want to tell you the safety rules at Hersey Retreat. First, as you've probably noticed, we are located on a large sandy bluff. The grassy fields out front end abruptly with steep sandy cliffs, and the bluff erodes easily. For your safety and for the environment, we ask you to stay away from the edge. We do not want to encourage further erosion. Kids, you must be accompanied by an adult if you are going down that way. There are posts up in the field, indicating where you should stop.

"Second, to get down to the beach, you can use either path that goes down around the bluff. They're well-marked. A nice walk would be going down one, walking along the beach around under the cliffs, and then back up the other path. It's passable at both high and low tide.

Third, no children are allowed to go down to the beach without an adult." She finishes, "Just briefly, the fourth rule is no smoking inside the lodge, and, please, put your cigarette butts in the cans provided. Any questions?" The group is quiet.

"We're a big group, but soon we'll all know each other. First, I'd like for everyone to go around and say their name and identify who you came with. If one of the family members will say where you come from, that would be just great. I'll go first. I'm Pat and I come from Bangor."

To Pat's left is one of our counselors. "I'm Ginny. I'm 17. I'm from Blue Hill, and I have diabetes." She looks to her left.

"I'm Brent Booth. I'm here with my wife Marjorie, my son Tate, and my daughter Susan who is diabetic. We are from Philadelphia."

"I'm Marjorie Booth."

"My name is Tate." He's really a cute kid, and I can just imagine all the fun he is going to have.

"I'm Susan Booth." Susan is soft spoken, quite serious, and her glasses take up most of her face.

Next to Susan is the mother from Port Clyde. I didn't catch her name at supper. She looks uncomfortable in her chair—it's a tight fit.

"My name is Lydia Stone from Port Clyde. I'm here with my son Kevin," who is sitting next to her, "and my daughter Cindy who's over there. Oh, and Kevin has had diabetes for five years."

"Kevin. I'm 11."

At this point I begin to wonder if I'll ever learn all the names. By the end of camp all of us will have shared much. But, at this point, there are so many faces. I need to focus on one special feature that will help me until I have a personal chance to talk with them. And it's even harder for the newcomers. They have all the anxiety of wondering if this will be worth it—a week's vacation dedicated to diabetes.

The boy sitting next to Kevin straightens. "I'm Peter McCabe, age 10, and I'm with my mom and dad and my sisters, Lucy and Abigail."

"Let me tell them where we are from! I'm Abigail. I am just eight and we are from Bar Harbor, Maine."

"I'm Mark McCabe, father of this tribe."

"And I'm Lisa McCabe, mother of this group."

There is a silence. The little girl, seated on Lisa's lap, is all of the sudden speechless. She had been chattering away. Lisa whispers in her daughter's ear. The little girl shakes her head. Her mother finally says, "Well, this is Lucy. She's four." The little girl buries her blond head in mom's shoulder, but only for a few seconds.

I have known the McCabe's for only six months. Peter came down with diabetes this past January. It was the coldest day of the year and they had trouble getting their car started to drive to Bangor. He stayed in the hospital for about six days for education. His mother, an X-ray technician, had a fairly good understanding of diabetes and had given shots before. Mark, a very supportive father, sometimes brings Peter to diabetes clinic. The two girls come, too. Little Lucy is not generally shy. This will soon change soon, I'm sure. Abigail wants to be a nurse when she grows up, so she is very interested in her big brother's problem.

Next to Lisa McCabe is a dark haired woman whose face is thin and drawn. "I'm Nancy Russell and this is my husband, Darryl, and my daughter, Becky." She has little expression.

"Darryl Russell. Glad to be here. We're from Medina, Ohio."

"My mother already told you who I am and I'm 12." There is a slight pause in introductions as we all note Becky's hostility.

The teenage girl who was at my table says, "I'm Cindy." She barely lifts her head.

"I'm Eddy Jelkepski from Lewiston, Maine. I was here seven years ago when I was 10. I'm really glad Pat and Dr. Mac chose me as a counselor."

"I'm Dr. MacCracken, Dr. Mac, occasionally Dr. Cracken, and to the adults, Joan. I live in Orono." As the years have gone by I've tried all sorts of names. I don't particularly like "Doc." The reason I like to be called "Dr. MacCracken" is twofold, I think.

First, from experience we learned that if I'm called "Joan," then the younger kids at the end of camp have no clue I'm a doctor. And I do think it is good for them to identify me as a nonthreatening, fun-loving person who also happens to be a doctor. And some kids still haven't known any women doctors.

Second, if they call me by my first name at camp, it is very likely that they will continue to call me that if they come to the office later. And that's very confusing for other clinic patients. So this is the solution we've reached, and it seems to work. The parents are able to use whatever they are comfortable with.

"My name is Jeffrey Peterson. I'm seven. I'm here with my mom and my brother Kyle. My dad couldn't come 'cuz of his new job."

"I'm Kyle. I'm eight. We come from Old Town, Maine."

"I'm Lucy Peterson." I've known this family for four years. Jeffrey has tried to be such a big boy about his diabetes. He has almost mastered the injection technique and is working hard to learn how to draw up the insulin, too. Lucy has rheumatoid arthritis, and her fingers are quite stiff, making it difficult for her to hold onto the syringe. I guess she's doing pretty well right now. Steve, her husband, told me during a clinic visit that she takes gold therapy injections once a month. Lucy, who never talks about her problems, is one of the most positive and energetic people I know. She's an inspiration.

"I'm Heather, the camp dietitian, from Milford. Sorry I was late, but my dog was hiding from me. I had to find him before I could leave." Heather is an integral part of our staff. She adds a great sense of humor along with her knowledge of nutrition.

The next camper doesn't look too happy to be here. He's a big guy with a red beard. Oh, yes, this is Sam, the first to arrive in the red Chevy truck. Pat told me a little bit about him. He has diabetes as does his daughter. I think her name is Emily. They have come with Sam's mother. I recall there was something tragic that happened to Emily's mother, but I can't remember exactly.

"Sam Wright from Houlton."

"I'm Pearl Wright, and this is Emily." She gives a loving squeeze to the little dark-haired, dark-eyed girl sitting on her lap. Emily couldn't be more than five years old. "She is my granddaughter, and Sam is my son." Emily remains mute.

"Well, we did it. Now does everyone know each other?" The crowd responds with giggles, coughs, and "no's."

Pat continues, "No? Well, now comes the fun." She pulls a very large ball of red yarn out of a brown paper bag . "The idea is to call out the name of someone and throw it to them while you hold on to the end. Try to pick other people besides your family. I'll start." She shouts, "Darryl," and throws the red yarn ball all the way across the room.

Darryl catches it, holds on to it as he looks around the room for a face he can put with a name. He's having a bit of trouble, but then spies Heather, whom he sat next to at supper. "Heather!" He tosses it underhanded in the right direction. The ball doesn't quite reach her but bounces on the floor first and rolls to her. Luckily, he remembers to keep hold of his end of the yarn.

Heather calls out, "Peter," and Peter, an athletic kid, catches it with no difficulty. Everyone is beginning to smile. This is fun. Imagine what the spider web will look like when we are done. Peter tosses the yarn to another camper.

I've always been amazed how this game works. I guess it is the auditory and visual components that help, as well as the repetition. What a fantastic feeling as the barriers begin to break down. Every year I think to myself, "Boy, I hope this works this time."

Abigail throws the yarn ball to her father, "Daddy," she screams.

Mark catches the ball and says, "My name is Mark, but you can all call me Daddy if you'd like." His warmth radiates from his face. He probably would be a good Daddy for the whole camp. One year we had only one father here along with single moms and women whose husbands couldn't or wouldn't come. That one Dad filled many needs for those campers.

Since then, Pat and I try to insist that if there is a dad in the family, he must come. That is our strong conviction, because we know how much fathers get out of this experience. But even with a firm decision, we just can't always have our way. We had hoped that Steve Peterson could come, but with his new job it was impossible this year. He is going to try to come to some evening activities. So we must adapt.

Mark looks around, pauses, and then calls, "Sam," and flings the ball all the way across the room. Sam has been sitting there very quietly. I think he has been listening. He grabs it with his large hands. He has no clue what the names of the remaining players are.

Heather, on his right, leans over, and suggesting someone. "Nancy," Sam says with little expression. He gently flips it to Nancy. With several more throws and assistance from Pat, the spider web is completed.

"We did it," everyone yells. We look at our artistic creation.

"Yep, we did, but now . . . ," and Pat leans over and reaches into her brown bag, "we need to do it faster." We groan. She grabs another roll of yarn, this one white. "Put down the first web, and we'll go faster with this one. Repeats are allowed, but try to throw it to someone new."

Pat shouts, "Mark."

Mark says," Kyle."

Kyle yells, "Peter." The new white yarn ball flies swiftly across the room. Back and forth it goes with names and faces becoming more and more familiar. The faster it goes, the more fun it is. There are a few hesitations. The two little girls, Emily and Little Lucy, try to play, too. With some assistance they catch on. After about two passes to everybody, I catch the ball and throw it to Pat.

"Well, I am very, very impressed with this group. You all have done a great job. Now, what we have done in the past is ask if anyone would like to volunteer to try and name everyone in the circle." There are groans from some campers.

Jeffrey's mother, Lucy, says, "I'll try." She looks to her left and begins. "Heather, Sam, Emily, Pearl, Pat, Ginny . . . ." She hesitates. "Don't tell me," she insists. "Oh, yes, Brent, Marjorie, Tate, Susan, Lisa."

"No, Lydia," corrects Lydia.

"Oh, sorry, Lydia, Kevin, Peter? Abigail, Mark." She again hesitates. "Lisa?" Lisa nods. "Lucy . . . ."

"Me, Little Lucy and you, Big Lucy," interrupts the little girl. Everybody smiles.

Big Lucy continues, "Nancy, Darryl, Becky, Cindy, Eddy, Joan, Jeff, and Kyle." We all applaud. I'm impressed.

Pat compliments, "Good job, Big Lucy. Would anyone else like to try?" We used to just go around in a circle and have everyone try it. But one year we found a mother who was so anxious about doing it. She had a learning disability and couldn't recall any more than about five or six names. She was very embarrassed when six and seven year olds were able to do it. She just had to say she just didn't want to try. Since then, we have asked for volunteers, and most folks have wanted to take the challenge. For those who don't try, just the multiple repetitions by others help.

Eddy successfully names everyone. Everyone applauds loudly. A perfect job from a guy who really wanted to learn all those names and faces. Hurray.

Several others try. Most of them do very, very well. Of course, we are all very impressed when Tate, the little six year old, says, "I think I can." He proceeds to list everyone correctly but trips a bit in saying "Dr. MacCracken." So he just says, "Doc," and goes on, completing the circle. Cindy, the teenage girl from Port Clyde, and Sam, our red bearded father, are the only ones, besides the two little girls, who don't try. No one pushes them.

During this whole time the kids have been great. But now some kids are getting fidgety. After meeting and naming so many new people, everyone could use a good night's sleep. I know I could.

"A couple of announcements before we go out in the hall for our bedtime snack," says Pat. "Because you are all sleeping under one roof, we have a curfew for noisy activities. No ping-pong, piano, or pool after 9 P.M. Unfortunately, sound carries upstairs all too well. Quiet conversations in the meeting room are fine. Parents can determine their own kids' lights out times, but if they stay up after 9, we request, for the sake of those who want to go to bed, that they are quiet."

"Heather, Pat, and I leave here around 9 and sleep in the white cabin at the end of the driveway. Ginny will be in the room at the top of the stairs, and Eddy is downstairs just left of the main door.

They can help you if you have any questions. If you need us in the middle of the night, one of them can come down and get us." Everyone smiles, hoping that no one will have to do that.

Pat continues, "The hall lights are left on so folks can find their way in the night. If you haven't already noticed, we have posted one bathroom upstairs for girls and one for boys. The showers are on the third floor, also labeled boys and girls, two stalls each."

Heather comments, "There will be crackers, milk, and juice in the refrigerator in the staff office if you need food in the night."

"What time is breakfast?" Kevin asks.

"The daily schedule of events will be posted on the board the night before. Breakfast every morning will be at 8 A.M. The wake up bell will be at 7 o'clock. We ask that everyone be quiet until 7. No ping-pong, piano, or pool before then. Any other questions?"

"Can we have our snack now, Pat?" Jeffrey asks.

"Sure, let's do it!" Pat says.

The kids charge out of the room, and the smell of the popcorn is heavenly. Ginny and Eddy, our counselors, give each camper a small brown paper bag of popcorn. Some apples, bananas, milk, and crackers are available.

Everyone stands around eating their popcorn. The younger boys, Kyle, Jeffrey, and Peter, play a little pool as they munch on their snack. They are getting along nicely. Cindy quietly plays the piano, and Little Lucy pounds a few additional notes. The older girl doesn't seem to mind.

I notice Susan, Tate's sister, washing her hands. She is about to check a blood sugar with her machine, which is neatly kept in a small green bag. As she waits for the digital reading to appear on her machine, she readies her pen to record the value on her flow sheet and on the chart, posted especially for her on the front bulletin board. Each child has his or her own chart for recording the blood sugar values.

With his pack of Camel cigarettes in his shirt pocket, Sam steps outside. Probably for a smoke. No one knows he has diabetes yet.

Pearl, his mother and a very attractive middle-aged woman, converses quietly with Pat, as Heather distracts Pearl's granddaughter, Emily. Heather asks the little dark-haired girl about the black stuffed bunny tightly tucked under her arm. I can only hope Sam will begin to feel more comfortable here. He certainly didn't mention his diabetes in the introduction circle. Pearl was sensitive not to say anything. We'll just have to see how he is going to handle this.

Nancy and Darryl approach me. Darryl's balding head and small chin remind me of my next door neighbor in Boston. Nancy, his wife, says nothing at first. Darryl speaks, "We are really happy to be here. We hope Becky will meet some nice friends and see that other kids have diabetes and get along with it." He looks around to be sure his daughter is out of earshot. She is over talking to Ginny, our counselor, at the popcorn machine. "We've really had a lot of trouble with her."

Now Nancy speaks, but in a soft voice. "Becky and I have been having some bad times lately. It seems that any suggestions I make are stupid and mettlesome. She's gotten so she hates testing. I think she actually writes down any number just to get me off her back. And she'd rather listen to her tapes than talk with me."

Nancy whispers, "We've heard that this camp works miracles—and we could sure use one."

"I'm flattered that news of our camp has traveled out to Ohio, but I'm afraid our successes have been exaggerated across the miles. But I'm sure our camp will give Becky some things to think about and I know she'll make some friends here. But miracles? Well, I don't know. She's talking to a good role model right now. Maybe Ginny will be able to help her." We all look over that way. The two girls are laughing. Maybe, just maybe.

By this time of night, I'm pretty tired. I'd guess everyone is ready for bed. Pat finishes her conversation with Pearl, and we head for the door. Some parents are rounding up their children to head to bed. Little Lucy melts in her father's arms as he carries her upstairs. We walk out the door, and Sam passes us. I say "Good night."

He replies, "Night." The lingering odor of cigarette smoke passes by. Hopefully, he's going to help Pearl put Emily to bed.

It's dark outside as Heather, Pat, and I walk to our cabin. The stars are beautiful. Away from the city lights, they are so much more brilliant. It's cool out, a great temperature for sleeping.

During the first five years of family camp we all slept in the main lodge. We shared rooms and lived together with everyone. It really wasn't too bad. Actually, the campers got a kick out of brushing their teeth with their doctor, and it certainly made us available at every moment. But with no rugs and no curtains, the main lodge is quite noisy.

We decided it would be better for us to have a little more privacy. Maybe we were just getting old. But with two or three counselors who are experienced with diabetes, (because they themselves have it) we feel comfortable leaving at 9 P.M. and returning at 7 A.M. And it has worked out well. I don't think the families have missed out on much. It's true I don't brush my teeth with them anymore. But, honestly, I think it has had a positive effect.

Once the parents get their kids settled down, some adults drift back downstairs to sit by the fire. Many nights they have talked late into the night, taking the opportunity to share some of their deepest feelings and fears. We aren't there to hear their words, and perhaps, without us, they open up even more. At least that's been true other years. We can only hope the sharing will happen here, too.

At the cabin, we collapse in the soft chairs and sofa. "So, what are you two creating this year?" I ask. For the past several years Heather and Pat have brought their arts and crafts with them. One year Heather was into making rugs. She called it her therapy.

Last year they were both weaving baskets. I marvel at their energy. During the school year they took night classes on basket weaving. Pat's children are grown and out of the home. Heather has no kids. I'm ready to go to bed after a day at work seeing patients, and then attending a soccer game or music lesson, helping with homework, and maybe finally paying some bills or opening some two-day-old mail. I can't imagine fitting basket weaving into my family's schedule.

"We are knitting this year," Heather replies. "I'm knitting a sweater for my dog and some little doggie booties."

Pat's daughter got married last year and is expecting a child at Christmas. She says, "I've decided to knit a green and red sweater with a Santa Claus face on the back. That way I don't have to worry about pink or blue." She smiles. Pat will be a wonderful grandmother. But, my God, she's younger than I am. I smile.

"Want a soda, Joan?" Heather asks.

"Sure, have any diet Pepsi?"

"Only, diet Coke," she replies.

"That's fine. But what would Ray Charles say?"

Heather laughs. She goes to the refrigerator, a nice convenience, and brings out three diet Cokes. She also brings out the Triscuits, and we start to munch.

"Well, this is going to be another challenging year, I'd say." Pat always is prone to the understatement. Usually, we stay up late talking about each family and our first impressions. But tonight we admit fatigue. And tomorrow will be another day.

Pat reviews tomorrow's events for us. Then she gets out the necessary supplies, while I stare at my list of campers. Six families, all new to each other. That's a challenge, right there.

Getting
to Know You

Monday morning. It's sunny and beautiful. The blue sky and ocean mirror one another. Not a cloud in the sky. The tide is in. No wind yet, but it usually picks up in the afternoon. The dew-covered fields glisten with rainbow reflections. The splendid lupine, pink, purple, and white, stand tall in the stillness. This Maine scene is etched in my mind and heart.

Pat's up and showers first. I'm next. Heather likes to sleep in. She's a morning person, she says, but we keep her up too late at night, so she can't get it together until after her first cup of coffee. We do like to tease her.

Pat and I walk over to the main lodge. Three kids are already up riding their bikes around the circular porch, an automatic highway for tricycles and Big Wheels. The larger bikes are a bit more dangerous. We could use a few of those mirrors that help you look around corners. But the kids never seem to worry about what's around the corner.

"Hi, Pat," says Jeff, as he peddles by.

"Looks like he's enjoying himself already today," I comment.

Almost everyone is downstairs, and it's only 7:15. They seem eager to get the week's activities started. The list of daily activities is on the bulletin board by the front door.

Special activities change from day to day, but there is a certain routine that is necessary for the life of a child with diabetes. The wake- up bell is 7 A.M. At 7:30 we try to gather and do blood sugar tests together. Insulin injections are given, and breakfast is at 8. After breakfast we have an educational activity. This morning the chart says "Get a Clue game," followed by "Food Groups," a break for snack, and then "Dietary Auction."

Next to the daily activity chart is the dishwasher schedule. Two adults and one child are assigned for breakfast and another group for dinner. Assigned dish washing encourages interaction— and gets the dishes done. The counselors do the lunch dishes.

Each person with diabetes has a blood testing chart posted on the bulletin board. We encourage them to fill it in. At first, some are upset about others seeing their blood glucose readings, but we try to show them that it will be an educational experience for all. Susan's and Peter's charts have results from last night. Otherwise, the charts are empty.

Kevin taps me on the shoulder. "What's a Dietary Auction?"

"Oh, you'll see after breakfast. It's quite an auction."

Pat watches some of the kids do their blood tests. There are many different brands of blood testing machines, and she must be knowledgeable about all of them. To obtain an accurate reading, the importance of good technique must be emphasized.

"Jeff, did you wash your hands first?" inquires his mother.

"Ooops, I forgot."

"Pat, do you have any extra strips; I've run out."

"Pat, will you show me how to use this meter? I don't like mine."

"Where do I record my result?"

Pat, our patient saint, handles each question one by one. Most of the kids are actually enjoying this activity, which is usually not such a pleasant time. Some kids claim testing is boring, too time-consuming, or just too painful.

Pearl is downstairs with Emily, who refuses to have her finger pricked. Her grandmother says it has been harder and harder to do a blood test because Emily fights her so much. "She says it really hurts. I feel so bad. Am I doing it right?" she asks Pat.

Pat looks at Emily's fingers, and the small dots of the lancet are located in the correct areas. We encourage folks to use the sides of the fingers and not the middle of the finger pads. But Emily's older model of blood pricker could be going a bit deeper than necessary. The newer models are adjustable for depth. Because she is so young and doesn't have tough skin, a light prick is all she needs.

Emily, let's try it with this newer one," Pat urges.

No, no," Emily cries and squirms.

Pearl says, "Maybe if we go upstairs, she'll let me do it." Emily grabs her grandmother's hand, and they go upstairs with the new finger pricker.

We have had many small children who do not like to have their fingers pricked or their insulin given in front of others. And we appreciate this. Usually after a day or so, when these strangers have become friends, they don't seem to mind anymore. But we don't push. Usually.

While this discussion was going on, the other children got their insulin shots. Some went upstairs to give or receive them. Others injected themselves in front of new friends. We try to have the kids take their shots about 20 to 30 minutes before the meal, but this doesn't always work out.

The bell rings over at the French House. "Tate, would you like to ring the bell here?" He jumps up on the bench. Barely reaching the string, he pulls it. Everyone gathers around to hear a few announcements from Pat. "On dish duty this morning—Kyle, Big Lucy, and Darryl. Morning activities will begin in the meeting room around 9. Let's go to breakfast."

All the kids, except Emily, run to the French House, as if they are starved. Some may be. The adults walk more slowly, enjoying the crisp morning air. At the end of the line Emily walks over with her grandmother on one side and her father Sam on the other.

As we all sit down for breakfast, I notice that the campers are a little more mixed in their seating arrangements. Peter, Jeff, and Kyle are all sitting together. Becky and Cindy are with Ginny in the other room. Otherwise, I guess, everyone is still with their parents. Pat, looking vibrant, stands with coffee cup in hand and sleepy Heather next to her. Pat looks over at me and announces that we sometimes like to sing a grace. "These are the words we use. It's the Johnny Appleseed song. 'Oh, the Lord is good to me, and so I thank the Lord, For giving me the things I need, The sun, the rain and the insulin, The Lord is good to me'." Everyone chuckles at our creativity. "Now, let's sing it." And we do.

Then, we all dive into breakfast, which today is one of my favorites; it's called "bird in a nest," one of Laurie's (the cook) specialties. It consists of a piece of bread with a hole punched out in the middle. Then, an egg is cooked right in the middle of the piece of bread. We eat toast, egg, and even the toasted holes. Usually, it's a hit with the campers. Of course, we also have fruit, juice, cereal, and yogurt available. Some of the older children with diabetes appear to know their meal plans for breakfast. A few kids pay no attention, eating what they want, while still others ask their mothers what they can have. Soon breakfast ends and all but the dishwashers, counselors, and staff leave the dining hall.

This sink is rather low," says Darryl, who bends way over to wash. He smiles as Laurie, our cook, who is five feet tall, tells him it was made especially for her. I offer him a stool to sit on. Over the years it's the only way I can wash and avoid major backaches.

Thanks, Doc," he says, as he sits. Eight-year-old Kyle does a great job drying while his mother works on the silverware. They all appear to be having a good time. Dish washing, though no one would initially believe it, is one of the best icebreakers. Somehow, strangers open up and become acquainted over the suds.

How long has Kyle had diabetes?" Darryl asks Kyle's mother.

"I don't have diabetes, my brother does!" insists Kyle. I hear the conversation continue as I check the counselors, who are wiping the tables and sweeping the floors. We've always had some extra help around to do the small kitchen jobs, but for the past two years we've chosen our counselors from older kids who attend our diabetes clinic. And it has been a big addition. I hope Ginny and Eddy will have a good time here. They are both great kids.

"Eddy, you left a crumb under this chair," I point to a speck of bread on the floor.

"Oh, so sorry!" Eddy jests, as he comes over to pick it up. I smile, giving him a little punch in the arm. We've known each other for seven years, ever since he first came here with his family. They're wonderful people. I know Eddy's upset about his little sister. Six months ago, Marie, who is a twin, developed diabetes. He really took it hard, as did the rest of the family. But I think it's better now. I need to talk to Eddy about it. There should be time this week.

"Dr. MacCracken, do you want me to get the art room ready for this afternoon's quiet hour? I couldn't find any paint up there," Ginny inquires. She will be a great help with art as she's very talented. In fact, I have a few of her paintings hanging in my office.

"When it comes to the organizational points here at camp, you need to ask Pat. She either knows where the paints are or has a different idea for the T-shirts and banners."

"OK," Ginny says, and we all head off for the main lodge.

Around 9 A.M., Peter asks to ring the bell to start the morning session. We all gather in the meeting room. Pat hands a jarful of pencils to Eddy and Ginny to distribute. Then, she hands out the Clue Sheets. This is another get-acquainted game that gets people talking. Some folks are good at names and faces, and others are shy and reserved. This activity forces more interaction.

I gaze at my paper.

Getting to Know Each Other

1. Carries nails and hammers to work
2. Loves kittens and bunny rabbits
3. Works with books for a living
4. Wants to be a nurse
5. Loves the color purple, any shade
6. Tells Downeast stories
7. Having a birthday this week
8. Wants to learn more karate
9. Wants to be a clown
10. Likes to sing and play piano
11. Likes squash (not the kind you eat)
12. Loves baseball
13. Met President Bush once
14. Likes to play with legos
15. Plays the clarinet
16. Loves to sing
17. Lived in Alaska once
18. Has read all Stephen King's books
19. Makes crafts out of lobster shells
20. Looks forward to 1994 World Cup Soccer
21. Wants a puppy dog
22. Wants to be a lawyer
23. Coaches kids soccer team
24. Enjoys reading a good book
25. Loves the Boston Red Sox
26. Loves her dog

Pat explains the task. "Everyone try and fill in the blanks by going around and asking, for example, 'Do you like to play legos?' If the answer is yes, then you write that person's name in the space. Then, that person can try to guess which is your clue. The clues were submitted on your camp registration form. If you don't know your clue, ask your mother or father; if they can't remember what clues they sent in, then ask me. Only I have all the answers. The first person to correctly fill in all the blanks wins a prize. Little Lucy and Emily can work with a parent."

Now the room is loud and wild as people wander around talking to one another. A few of these clues I already know, but you are supposed to talk to people to verify the clue.

Tate comes over to me and says, "Do you want to be a lawyer?" I laugh aloud. Someone put him up to this. That is too perfect a question. Besides, at age six, he probably can't even read. I glance over at Heather, and she has a huge smile on her face. She's a card.

"That's one for you, Heather," I shout in her direction. She laughs.

"No, Tate, I don't want to be a lawyer. Do you want a puppy dog?"

"No, we already have two goldens."

"Do you want to learn more karate?"

"Yep, sure do," he replies as he takes a defensive posture. I recognize this only because we always have one kid here at camp who knows karate and usually give us a demonstration.

Becky, standing within earshot, quickly writes Tate's name down for clue number 8. She is working the crowd quite well and looks determined to win. It's good to see her get into something.

Loving the racquet game of squash, I figure I need to meet this other squash player. By deduction, because there are hardly any squash courts in Maine, I figure it must be Darryl from Ohio or Brent from Philadelphia. I suppose it could be Marjorie or Nancy, but neither looks too athletic. I walk over to Brent, the most obvious choice. "Want to play squash someday?" I ask.

"Do you play? Where is the nearest court?" he jokes.

"In Orono, at the University."

"Well, you'll have to come to Penn sometime for a match."

"That sounds like fun." I write Brent in my number-11 spot.

And everyone else is doing the same thing. It's fun seeing the mingling going on. I overhear Jeff and Eddy discussing the sad fate of the Boston Red Sox in the 1990 playoffs against the Oakland A's.

I interrupt and find out that Eddy's first love is the Red Sox. I suppose it's obvious because he hardly ever takes off his blue baseball hat with the red "B." Jeff loves the game too and has just been moved up from T-ball to little league.

The game goes on. I need to find out who met President Bush. His summer compound is in Kennebunkport, Maine, so I suppose it could be anyone in the room, but I've narrowed my choices considerably by filling in all but four spaces. My remaining clues are having a birthday this week, has read all Stephen King's books, loves to sing, and met President Bush. Let's see, what names do I not have on my sheet. Now, this is hard because, if you don't know their names, you have to see what faces you don't have on your sheet.

"Dr. MacCracken, I have only two spots to fill in," says Becky.

"That's great, and how can I help you?"

"Well, either you have met President Bush or you want to be a clown."

"Well, I've met Senator Mitchell and Senator Cohen, our Maine Senators, but I've never met the President."

"So you must want to be a clown," she proclaims with glee. "And it must be that boy over there who met Bush. What's his name?" she asks me.

"Oh, no, you have to speak with him to get his name." She runs over and interrupts Kevin who is interrogating Darryl, Becky's father.

"What is your name?" she inquires forcefully.

"Kevin."

"I've got it, Pat. I've got all the names."

"Good job, Becky. Bring your sheet over so I can check the answers, and we'll give the others a few more minutes. You were pretty quick," Pat adds. I wonder how many campers she actually spoke with. But it's just a game.

Sam isn't too active in this game. He waits for people to come around and tells them he is a carpenter. He makes a slight attempt at filling in his paper, but most of the answers come from Pearl's paper. She appears to be enjoying this game.

I find out it is Pearl who is having a birthday this Thursday. She is going to be 50. Her strawberry blond hair and her spunk make her a young-looking grandmother.

Pat says, "OK, we better call it quits on this game now. I hope you've had an opportunity to find out more about each other. I know I'm curious to hear about Kevin's meeting with the President. Kevin, would you tell us how that happened?"

"Well, he was going out to Monhegan for a meeting with the Prime Minister of Canada to talk over off sea fishing rights. I was in a crowd of people standing around the special boat that was going to take them out. When he walked by, I stretched out my hand. He turned and shook it and asked my name."

"Were you scared?" asked Jeff.

"Nah, just surprised."

"That makes you famous," adds Kyle. Kevin smiled.

"Well, this morning, Becky is our winner. For her we have a little prize." Pat reaches into the bag on the piano and pulls out a pink T-shirt with the American Diabetes Association, Maine Affiliate, logo. Becky takes the prize but doesn't look too pleased. "You can all check with her answer sheet if yours isn't complete. I'll hang it on the board.

The answers . . . .
1. Carries nails and hammers to work: Sam
2. Having a birthday this week: Pearl
3. Loves kittens and bunny rabbits: Emily
4. Likes squash (not the kind you eat): Brent
5. Works with books for a living: Marjorie
6. Loves the color purple, any shade: Susan
7. Wants to learn karate: Tate
8. Likes to sing and play piano: Cindy
9. Makes crafts out of lobster shells: Lydia
10. Met President Bush once: Kevin
11. Plays the clarinet: Becky

12. Loves to sing: Nancy
13. Has read all Stephen King's books: Darryl
14. Looks forward to World Cup Soccer: Peter
15. Wants to be a nurse: Abigail
16. Wants a puppy dog: Lucy
17. Coaches kids soccer team: Lisa
18. Tells Downeast stories: Mark
19. Loves baseball: Jeff
20. Likes to play with legos: Kyle
21. Enjoys reading a good book: Lucy
22. Loves the Boston Red Sox: Eddy
23. Wants to be a lawyer: Ginny
23. Lived in Alaska once: Pat
24. Loves her dog: Heather
25. Wants to be a clown: Dr. Mac

Most of Monday we dedicate to dietary concerns. It is perhaps the least threatening of all the topics we'll cover. Besides, it gives us another day to get to know the families and for them to get to know us and each other. Monday is the start of the formal educational process but we don't ever get too formal.

In the hall is a table with lots of literature on diabetes including a collection of reprints that parents have found useful in previous years. Some articles are more scientific than others. While many parents enjoy these detailed articles, others need less technical writing. We've also had some parents who could not read. These folks need one-on-one education. Several books about diabetes are also available.

Heather brings no less than five cookbooks as well as reprints of her favorite recipes. We usually try some here. *Grilled Cheese at Four O'Clock in the Morning* is a great book for kids. During the camp week, Pat sometimes reads it as a bedtime story. The adults enjoy it too.

Larry Pray's *Journey of a Diabetic* has been popular with many parents and older campers. Larry first came to our camp as a visiting author. He liked the idea of our family camp and returned first for a few days. Later, as a staff member, he stayed the entire week with his twin sons. Unfortunately, his job as a full-time minister in Minnesota has prevented him from joining us for the last several years. We miss his great banjo playing and his first-hand diabetes experience. Several American Diabetes Association publications are included on the table with several copies of the ADA's *Diabetes Forecast* magazines, which some of our families here are not familiar with.

In addition to the book table, Pat prepares a folder for each family, which they find in the their rooms on arrival. This includes schedule of events and useful handouts and reprints on such topics as sick days, exercise, artificial sweeteners, prevention of low blood sugar, what your teacher should know, the *Somogyi phenomenon* * (lows to highs), and stress.

In their rooms, the families find some diabetes supplies, contributed by various drug companies. These companies are very generous in helping us obtain blood glucose strips, urine test strips, extra insulin, etc. A few of our camp families have been in great need of these supplies, which take a big chunk out of a family's budget. Insurance companies vary in their coverage of diabetes supplies, and some families have no insurance.

Heather is ready to start her session. "Kids, pull some chairs up to the front near the board here. Your parents can sit around the outside," she instructs. All the children except little Lucy move up to the front. Emily is now sitting on Ginny's lap and seems quite content. Ginny has been trying to make friends with Emily. Cindy and Becky sit together.

"Heather, when is the auction?" asks Kevin who has been waiting for the auction since before breakfast.

"After snack. But first we need to find out how much you smart kids know about nutrition."

"What's nutrition?" shouts Tate. His mother Marjorie is not nearby but looks displeased with his interruption.

"It's all about food and what your body needs to be healthy.

Words in italics are defined in the glossary at the back of this book.

Now, who knows the basic food groups?" Hands go up in the young audience.

"Fruit," says Jeff. Heather writes it on the white poster board.

"Spaghetti," calls out Kyle, not wanting to let his brother be the only responder.

"Kyle, do you know what food group spaghetti would be in?" Heather asks. A quizzical look appears on Kyle's face. Eddy, who is seated next to him, leans over and whispers.

"Carbo–hydrates," Kyle says with a big smile.

"Right, let's call it breads for the discussion. So, we have Fruits, Breads, what else do we eat?"

"Protein," says Becky.

"Protein. What would that include?"

"Ah, I think that would be meat," Becky adds.

"Good, Becky."

"And eggs," shouts Peter.

"And cheese," adds Susan, who has been holding her hand up high for some time but finally in desperation just calls out.

"You guys are really hot this morning," Heather comments.

"I'm thinking of another group of foods some of you may not like."

"Vegetables," says Abigail, who has been amazingly quiet.

"Abigail, name me three vegetables."

"Carrots, beans, and . . . "

"Broccoli," says Tate, with a pleased smile.

Now the kids are getting into it. All ten are listening fairly well. They are having fun and possibly learning at the same time. Little Lucy has been wandering in and out of the room. She has been gone a few minutes, and her mother Lisa goes to check.

The other parents are enjoying watching their kids perform. It's encouraging to listen to their children talk about foods. Someday all these kids will be on their own and need to know what they should eat. The burden of meal planning in a family with diabetes is just that—a burden, especially until you learn a little flexibility.

Many new parents get into a rut of feeding the children the same meals and snacks. Many parents complain that the spontaneity of meals is gone. Most of the time it's the mothers who complain of the energy it takes to feed their child what he or she is supposed to eat.

The dietitians have worked out what they call exchanges (others call them choices). It is a way to teach the food groups. But, actually, it's just a healthy, balanced, consistent yet varied diet. In reality, most Americans don't eat healthy, balanced, consistent yet varied meals. So, when diabetes enters a family's life, the typical American family's meals will have to change. And in some families that's a major adjustment.

It's enlightening to talk to kids with diabetes. Most get used to the shots and the finger sticks. Whereas folks without diabetes would claim it would be the injections two to four times a day they would hate the most, the people with diabetes on the whole will tell you it is the inability to eat anything you want that's the greatest burden. *(see Carbohydrate Counting in Glossary)

This really is an important point to keep in mind. For adolescents being different because you can't eat the hot fudge sundae or the huge 32-ounce Slurpee is a drag. Some of the children who have had diabetes since they were very young have known no other way. But the teenager, who one day eats everything and anything and the next day is told he or she has diabetes and will have to eat differently, has a harder time adjusting, I think.

Heather continues, "Susan's right. Milk is another food group. It has a combination of carbohydrate, protein, and fat, so we put it into its own group. We break foods down into six groups: milk, vegetables, fruits, breads, meats, and fats. If you don't already know how many of each group you are supposed to eat, I'll go over that with you and your parents this week. Who has heard the word 'Exchanges' used with their meal plan?" About half the kids raise their hands.

"You can use the word exchanges or choices. During this week, I'll have a piece of paper on your dining room table that lists what exchanges are represented in the meal. If you kids or parents have questions during the meals about where the foods fit, just ask me. "It's now 10:15. Let's take a break, stretch, have a snack if you need one, and then come back in ten minutes for the dietary auction."

The children push back their chairs and run out of the room. On the coffee table in the hallway are crackers and juice. Most of the kids, whether they have diabetes or not, are interested in a snack. Kevin helps himself to three crackers and lots of peanut butter.

"Kevin, Dr. Winters told you you don't need a morning snack," says his mom.

"Ah, Mom, I'm hungry."

"Just go play." Lydia heads upstairs for a little break.

"Dad, should I have a snack?" Susan asks her father Brent.

"You have been relatively inactive this morning, Susan. And your blood sugar was a bit high this morning.

"It was 130. Maybe I should just skip it this morning."

"Sure."

Heather, Pat, and I try not to make recommendations for the first few days of camp. We really feel it's a good idea to just observe in the beginning, to see how each family handles their own diabetes.

There are many ways to skin a cat, and it is presumptuous to assume that we always know the best way. Long ago I learned how important it was to listen to the parent and the child. Diabetes is a variable disease. And there are few hard and fast rules that work for all people. I guess that is one of the most frustrating things about the disease—and perhaps the most challenging.

During the dietary auction I just sit in the back of the room and enjoy the fun. Pat and Heather started this about three or four years ago, I think. It is a participatory game, and everyone gets involved.

"Come one, come all to the Diet Auction. Come and bid on the price. Who can guess the price according to calories?" Pat starts off in her effervescent way. "You've got your money, now let's start the bidding. Who can bid the closest to the correct calorie count on these foods? Little ones, your parents can assist."

Pat and Heather hold up the first item for bid. Actually, the items are drawn on a large poster board.

"How much will you give me for ten tablespoons of cream cheese? Do I hear fifty?"

"Fifty."

"One hundred," calls Jeff.

"Ten hundred," shouts Tate.

"Six hundred," guesses Susan.

"One thousand," calls Kevin.

"How many say one thousand?" Several hands go up. "Sold, for one thousand dollars." Kevin smiles.

"For our second item we have three chocolate cup cakes."

"O-O-Oh, seven thousand."

Pat points to another raised hand. "Four hundred." She points to another raised hand.

"Nine hundred."

"Eight hundred."

"How many say eight hundred? How many say nine hundred? The nines have it. Our next item is three hundred radishes."

Emily says, "I love radishes."

"Sixty," guesses Kyle.

"One hundred," says Jeff. He seems to like that number.

"Two hundred and fifty," Peter guesses.

"Sold for two hundred and fifty."

Heather holds up a picture of seven heads of broccoli. "Seven heads of broccoli. What will you give me?"

"Nothing!" shouts Kevin.

"Maybe that's why President Bush shook your hand," says Mark. "I'll give you two hundred, Heatha'." Mark seems to have decided that he'll play up his Maine accent. Heather gets a kick out of it.

"Anyone else have a bid for seven heads of broccoli?"

"Can we put butter on it?" asks Big Lucy.

"Not this time. Going once . . . going twice . . . sold to Mark for two hundred."

Several more items go up for bid. These include 6 pancakes with one teaspoonful of butter and a tablespoon of maple syrup, 4 tablespoons of butter, 12 large carrots, 3/4 of a cup of gravy (ugh), 5 small potatoes (no gravy) and 60 mixed nuts. Almost everyone is participating. The little kids love the high numbers and more enticing foods. Some of the mothers, like Marjorie and Nancy, try be more precise. I hear one of them multiplying four times one hundred and twenty five and then guessing five hundred. Her voice is just another number in the excitement of the dietary auction.

After the bidding calms down and the items are finished, Heather holds up the list of winning guesses next to the items listed. The guesses range from seventy to seven thousand for the pancakes with butter and syrup on top.

Heather says, "We played a little trick on you all. These all are worth approximately the same number of calories." She smiles and a few in the audience boo. "They are all equal to about five hundred calories."

I overhear Nancy comment to Marjorie, "Three hundred radishes is quite a bit. So each radish must be just under two calories. Too bad Becky doesn't like them."

Pat announces that it's time to check blood sugars, and then it will be lunch time. Folks drift out to the center hall where the blood testing equipment is. Kevin, Peter, and Susan go right to the table. Abigail is there too, trying to help out as a good nurse should. Emily goes upstairs with Pearl. Becky argues with her father. Probably, she just doesn't want to test. She never tests at lunchtime Nancy told me.

The counselors, Ginny and Eddy, quickly do their tests, record them, and hurry off to the French House to set up for lunch. Cindy sits by the piano and softly plays. Little Lucy accompanies her. Outside, Brent and Mark talk as Jeff, Kyle, and Tate kick a soccer ball around them. Sam stands aside having a smoke. The mothers surround Heather and must be discussing various dietary issues.

"Pat, I don't feel very good," says Susan. I walk over to the testing table. Susan has just pricked her finger and is getting ready to place it on the blood testing strip. Pat and I notice she has a white rim around her mouth and nose and is a bit sweaty. Her finger shakes as she applies the drop. She takes off her glasses and sits down.

Pat goes into the office and returns with a glass of orange juice. "Here, drink this, Susan. You are probably a bit low. Did you have a snack this morning?"

Marjorie comes over as she notices the small commotion. "She skipped her snack this morning because Brent thought she was too high at breakfast. Maybe that wasn't such a good idea. She was pretty active during the dietary auction."

At that moment the digital reading on Susan's machine shows 42. This low blood sugar undoubtedly is making her feel sick. She finishes the orange juice and requests a little more. Pat gets her a little more. The color in her face begins to return.

Luckily, the bell from the French House rings, so we can all head over for lunch. Marjorie, Susan, and Pat walk hand in hand over to the French House. The rest of the kids run. Holding on to the big banister and to Pearl's hand, Emily comes quickly down the stairs. She runs after the others. Pearl and I slowly walk to lunch. She wants a little time to talk with me in private.

The afternoon is sunny. A gentle breeze from the south is moist and warm. We might be in for some rain tonight. Pat and I retreat to our cabin after lunch. It is quiet hour until two. At least that's the idea. Families can go for walks on the beach, fly kites, or enjoy the luxury of an afternoon siesta. Ginny is in the art room on the third floor to help anyone with a project. This week we're making our own designs on T-shirts. Rest hour is a time to take a break.

Pat looks at me and instantly knows there's something on my mind.

"What's the matter?" she asks.

"I'm afraid we've got a problem."

"It's Sam, isn't it?" Pat doesn't miss much, though I suppose this time anyone could have guessed. Sam has not really jelled with the other campers. He came to the group session, but said very little. He smokes almost every chance he gets. Some years we've had lots of smokers, but this year only Sam smokes. He is younger than the other fathers and less educated. And he is obviously depressed.

"He wants to leave."

"Did he tell you that?" asks Pat.

"No, his mother told me on the way to lunch. Pearl says he plans to leave in the morning. He'll take Pearl and Emily, too."

"Well, Joan, we've had this happen before. Remember a few years ago the Littons were going to leave Wednesday morning. And remember Paul and Edith were going to go Monday morning after only being here less than twenty-four hours. But they all stayed—and had a good time, too. Are you going to try to convince him to stay?"

"I've got to try. I've had pretty good luck before at this. But, I have a feeling this one isn't going to be easy."

Pat puts her hand on my shoulder and says, "I know you can do it."

I shake my head. "This is going to be tough."

"Maybe I should tell you what I know about Sam. We didn't get a chance to talk about it last night."

"Any info would help, I'm sure." I'm not looking forward to this confrontation. But this is part of the job, a wrenching and mentally exhausting part of the job.

Pat begins, "Sam was 16 when he developed diabetes. He was living with his parents at the time and was a sophomore in high school in a town just north of Houlton. He got his diabetes education from an old general practitioner, who started Sam on one shot a day of intermediate-acting insulin. And he's still on one shot.

Anyway, at first Pearl says he was pretty good about checking his urine for sugar but that only lasted about a year. Sam usually felt OK so he gave up checking. Pearl says he got this girl, Rachel, pregnant when he was 18. He loved her and decided to get a job with his stepfather, who is a builder. He wanted to get married and keep the baby."

Pat continues. "Rachel got a job in a beauty salon, and Sam started to work. They lived upstairs in an apartment above Ollie, the stepfather, and Pearl. Pearl says Rachel was good for Sam. She made him take much better care of his diabetes. Rachel used to say to him, "I want you around for a long, long time." The baby was born seven months after the wedding. Emily was a jewel of a baby, and Rachel and Sam were very happy parents. Ollie and Pearl were so happy to have a little granddaughter. Pearl's other two sons, who are older, aren't married. One is in the Navy and the other has moved to Florida."

"When did Emily get diabetes?"

"When she was three, she started to lose weight and pee all the time. Pearl wondered about diabetes and asked Rachel to get her checked. The doctor checked her and said she had diabetes but it wasn't too bad yet. That night Rachel, Ollie, and Pearl met Sam when he came home from work. He couldn't believe it. Pearl said Sam just sat there and cried. He kept sobbing, 'It's all my fault. She got it from me. It just isn't fair.' None of them could comfort him. He refused to go to the hospital.

"He let Rachel get all the education, and he refused to give Emily any shots. He didn't want anything to do with her diabetes and he stopped taking care of his. Rachel took complete care of Emily's diabetes. She hardly ever asked for help from Pearl. One night, though, Rachel had to go out to a beautician training course. Sam was out. Pearl and Ollie were babysitting for a few hours. On the way home Rachel's car skidded on an icy turn. It flipped, and smashed into a tree. Rachel was killed instantly."

"Oh, God. That is horrible." Pat's eyes are moist.

"So, it's been about eighteen months since Rachel died. Sam is still working as a carpenter for Ollie. They all live together now. Pearl has tried to do the best she can for Emily. Sam loves her very much but just can't deal with her diabetes."

"Did Pearl say anything about how he's handling Rachel's death?"

"Ollie, his stepfather, got Sam to go to a counselor in Houlton. Ollie's first wife died of breast cancer about fifteen years ago, and he still remembers the pain. Sam seems to be working that out —as best as anyone can, but the diabetes hasn't made things easier."

"Well, we really ought to be able to help this family. Emily needs some joy, Pearl needs some support, and Sam needs some love, hope, and good friends. But we can't help them if they leave."

We, They, and Goldie Locks

Meeting with only the parents for the afternoon, Heather teaches nutrition and more specific meal planning. The mothers always have many questions about recipes, school lunches, artificial sweeteners, and such. The fathers listen and probably learn more than they've ever known about food. I think sometimes it gives them a greater understanding of and appreciation for what their wives have tried to juggle.

Many issues come up with meal planning and family choices. Some families elect to change the way everyone eats in the household when one member gets diabetes. That sure makes it easier for the cook. But many parents or siblings are not willing to deprive themselves of the junk food that most American families eat.

At camp we hear debates among the campers. "They [the people with diabetes] are going to have to face the fact that sweet foods exist in the outside world. They will need to learn their own self discipline. So we do have candy and cookies in the house for the others. It isn't fair to punish the other kids." Others say, "It's too much of a temptation to have that kind of food around. I just don't buy it. The rest of us don't really need it anyway. We all eat better because of our child's diabetes."

For each family there are compromises that are made. "Our daughter goes over to her friend's house for sweets." One mother admitted she was a candy freak and would just stop at the local store for a candy bar when she had no kids with her. "I know it is wrong, but I just can't help it."

Timing of meals can also be big problem. Now, some Maine families eat at 5 o'clock sharp, no matter what; it's been done that way for generations. But other families run into problems like Little League games or hockey practices or irregular work schedules. For many it is not easy to set the time consistently.

What if my child won't eat? What if he hates milk? How can I get the calcium into her? I need new ideas for snacks. How much diet soda can he safely have? Are Instant Breakfasts OK? These and many more questions are brought to Heather for comment and advice. And she does a great job.

Today, Heather is holding the session outside in the sun. The parents look relaxed. What a place for education. The questions start immediately.

My job this afternoon is to walk and talk with the siblings, the ones without diabetes. This year that includes Cindy, Kyle, Abigail, Tate, and little Lucy. Tate and Kyle have been having a great time playing hide and seek with Eddy. The main lodge has loads of nooks and crannies for hiding. Eddy and I gather all the kids together.

With little Lucy on my shoulders, we head down to the beach for a bit of exploration. Just as a precaution, I take some raisins in my pocket for Eddy, in case he is not carrying a source of quick energy. The other kids, even though they don't have diabetes, will probably enjoy a snack on the beach.

The tide is out, so there are many tide pools to explore. Lucy wants down as soon as we get to the beach. She stops to pick up a small white shell. The two sisters slow up, picking up more shells and jabbering together. Cindy walks next to me. She hasn't said much so far. Behind her unkempt hair is a delicate face with attractive eyes.

"Cindy, I have been listening to you play the piano. Have you taken lessons?" I realize that is a dumb question. How could her mother afford piano lessons.

"No, but I have a friend who takes lessons, and she tries to teach me. I practice with her after school."

"You like to sing, too? "

"Yeah, I love to sing. Mom lets me sing in the church choir."

"I hope you'll sing for us in our talent show."

"I've been practicing some songs from the Sound of Music. Our town is going to put on a summer production and I want to try out, but I'm not sure my mom will let me."

"Well, you can warm up on us Friday. It'll be a friendly audience." She smiles. If only I could get her to pull that hair back.

Eddy, Tate, and Kyle are skipping rocks. A great pastime. Tate's stones are too big, and he doesn't quite have the throwing angle right. Eddy tries to show him, and Kyle, who seems to find all the smooth and round stones, gives Tate a few "good" ones.

"How has Kevin's diabetes affected your life, Cindy?" I thought I'd try the direct approach. This camp is for the siblings, too. Sometimes they feel pretty left out, even discriminated against. Some siblings are mean and angry, while others are helpful and understanding. Some may appear oblivious. But all like to be heard.

"My mom doesn't like me. It's almost like she blames his diabetes on me. I'd nothing to do with it. She gets so worried about him that she doesn't have any time for me. And, recently, because of Lou, Kevin's been in the hospital a lot."

"Who's Lou?"

"He's my mom's new boyfriend. She wants to marry him."

"How does he cause Kevin to be in the hospital?"

Cindy flips some sand in the air with her foot. "Kevin hates him. He doesn't want Mom to get married. He likes it just him, me, and Mom. So, he figures if he gets sick a lot, Lou won't want to be in this family, and if Kevin has to be in the hospital, Mom won't have much time to be with Lou. I think Kevin eats extra, and I know that more than once he has not even taken his shot."

"Skipping insulin shots is pretty serious, Cindy. Have you tried to talk to Kevin?"

"You think an 11- year-old brother would consider listening to his older sister?"

"I see your point. Does your mother know Kevin is not taking his insulin?"

"I doubt it."

"So, you haven't told her?"

"She wouldn't believe me if I did!" She kicks some more sand.

"Do you like Lou?"

"He's OK. Mom is much nicer when he is around, and happier, too. I think she's been lonely for a long time. It isn't easy raising two kids on your own."

"That's for sure."

"Lou has a steady job of lobstering and makes good money. It wouldn't be so bad to live in a bigger house and be able to buy new clothes. I hate that thrift shop. And maybe if Mom were happier, she'd like me better."

"Maybe your mom just doesn't realize how you feel and doesn't realize she's giving so much attention to Kevin. When Kevin goes into the hospital, he takes your mom away from Lou, but also takes her away from you. We need to see if we can help Kevin realize that playing with his diabetes is dangerous and not really going to help the problem. I'll see what we can do."

"Good luck," she says with a skeptical note.

"Cindy, you keep practicing your songs. I'm signing you up for the Talent show, OK?

"I'll see."

The two sisters fill their pockets and mine with shells. We all start to walk around the bluff. Eddy, Kyle, and Tate walk a little ahead. We come to a big tide pool. The colors on the rocks below the water are so vibrant. The very small plants and plankton move ever so slightly, while the baby shrimp dart around.

"I've got one!" yells Kyle, and he holds up his crayfish. They look like small lobsters.

"He's big," says Abigail.

"Let me see! Let me see!" cries Little Lucy.

Time flies as we all explore and search for sea treasures. My plastic bag bursts with unusual shells and special rocks—the flattest, the whitest, the roundest.

Cindy and Eddy are talking and walking ahead with Lucy, Abigail, and Tate.

"Kyle, can I just ask you a question or two?"

"Sure, what about?"

"Jeff's diabetes. Does it cause you any problems?"

"No, but it's hard on my mom. She sometimes can't get her fingers working right. They get real stiff. Jeff and I try to help her then. If he didn't have diabetes, we wouldn't have to take the time out to check his blood and give his shots. Sometimes, we're busy building a great lego castle, and Mom interrupts us for his test. But he comes back pretty quick."

"So, you and Jeff pretty much do everything together?"

"Well, he gets to go to Toys'R'Us after his blood test and I don't, but Dad takes me ice fishing and occasionally bowling. Just me and him. He says I'm older and need some special times, too. Jeff came fishing with us once, and that was fun too. We each got two strikes. Dad got five!" This kid is great. I'd say that his mom and dad have made things pretty even. At least, it seems like that to Kyle. But it's probably true, knowing those two. I can't think of two more sensitive and loving folks.

"Should we catch up with the others?"

"Let's race," he says, as he takes off down the beach. I have to do a bit more than jog to catch up with him.

As we approach the others, I say, "You win."

"Well, I had a head start." We both smile.

Eddy has located a pocket of the natural clay, and Abigail, Tate, and Cindy are digging for some. Little Lucy doesn't like the gooey mess, yet. The blue-gray clay lies just under the sand in pockets. Along the bank of the cliff there is also a cache. This is a favorite project. The soft clay is very moldable. Tate brings me a pancake with his hand print in it.

"Good job, Tate," I say. "Anyone want a raisin?" I hold up the box. Little Lucy puts her tiny hand out. "Me, please." Now, that's a well-trained kid. I give her several, and she eats them one by one. The others wash the clay off their hands. The tide is coming in now, so the water isn't too far away. Eddy pulls out two granola bars to split. He tells me that ever since the time he collapsed on third base during the Little League playoffs, he always carries some food, just in case he starts feeling hungry. The other kids join us on the log and enjoy our snack.

These quiet moments are ones to treasure at camp. Even the kids who are always on the go enjoy listening to the waves and the seagulls. The wind is increasing. The gulls ride the wind currents. They appear motionless, not going anywhere, a seemingly effortless flight.

"We better head back now. It's getting on towards 4 o'clock."

"Can we take some clay back with us?"

"Sure." We head back up a wooded path that leads to the big fields and the main lodge.

From this southwest viewpoint we spy the main lodge, a dark green mansion with white trim. It sits high on the bluff, surrounded by beautiful grassy fields. As the wind gusts bend the long grasses in sporadic waves, I catch the scent of freshly cut grass. Somebody has just cut the path in the field and enlarged our baseball diamond. Wild blueberry bushes, scattered throughout, will bear fruit later this summer.

Approaching the retreat, I see that Heather and the parents are still talking. That's almost two hours of questions. She'll be ready for a break. Pat and the other kids are nowhere to be seen. Pat was planning on making some videos with the kids with diabetes. Maybe they're still working on it.

We hear thunder on the stairs. The other kids pour down from the third floor, their likely studio. The actors and actresses simultaneously tell us what they've been doing. Pat looks enthusiastic.

Finally, the parents break up their dietary session. Heather comes in and heads for the water fountain. Her face is sunburned. Everyone just relaxes now. Sam walks down the driveway with his cigarette.

At supper there is more mingling and chatter. I'd guess everyone knows everyone now. We've only been together 24 hours. Sam sits with his mother and his daughter Emily, who sits next to her new playmate, Little Lucy. Mark and Lisa, Lucy's parents, help serve the two little girls.

Pat and I take the two chairs at the other end of the table. Occasionally, Pat and I sit together. I can see the little girls playing with their mashed potatoes and peas. The chicken breasts are untouched on their plates. The meal is good. I'd certainly never complain. Just the luxury of having food prepared for me is heaven enough. Cooking is not my favorite pastime.

Pat makes her announcements. "At 7 o'clock, we'll gather in the meeting room and have a special show, compliments of the KiWiDi Video Company."

"What's KiWiDi?" asks Abigail.

"We'll tell you tonight," Peter and Kevin say at the same time.

Pat continues, "And after that we may have time for a little group singing to warm us up for the campfire on Wednesday. Dishwashers, do you know who you are?

"Yep," says Lydia.

"Do I have to?" says Becky, the difficult teen from Ohio. With encouragement from Ginny, Becky slowly rises.

"Who's the third lucky one," says Pat. She looks at the list posted on the door by the kitchen. "And the winner is . . . Marjorie!"

41

Tate laughs. "Mommy's got the dishes, Mommy's got the dishes." Everyone leaves but the lucky three and Eddy and Ginny, who laugh as they sweep the floors and wipe the tables.

At 7, Kevin calls out, "Ring the bell, Peter, it's time for the show." The TV and video machine are set up in the meeting room. Peter and Kevin have arranged the chairs in rows. Some of the kids sit on the floor in front of the screen.

Becky, Susan, Kevin, Peter, and Jeff stand before the group. "Emily, come on up here," says Susan. She reaches out her hand, and Emily, with a smile, comes up front, too.

"Welcome, ladies and gentlemen. We are the KiWiDi Video Company. That stands for Kids With Diabetes. Tonight we want to show you a special video we made this afternoon. So, sit back in your chairs. We hope you will enjoy this." Peter is a very well spoken 10- year-old. Maybe he should go into showbiz.

Kevin turns out the lights and Ginny, the production manager, hits the button. All eyes are on the screen.

First, we hear about the story of Goldie Locks and the Three Bears. Kevin plays Papa Bear, Becky plays Mama Bear, Jeff plays Baby Bear and Susan plays Goldie Locks. The bears leave their home, and Goldie Locks walks in. On the table in front of her are three bottles of insulin.She picks up Papa Bear's insulin, "This one is too long acting." She picks up Mama Bear's insulin. "This one is too short acting." She reaches for the third bottle. "This one is just right. It's intermediate-acting insulin." And she gives herself a shot.

Later, the three bears return. "Who's been using my insulin?" says Papa Bear.

"Who's been using my insulin?" asks Mama Bear.

"Someone's been using my insulin—and used it all up!"says Baby Bear.

As they look around, they see Goldie Locks asleep on the bed. They try to arouse her, but she's very groggy. "We better give her some honey if she used up all your insulin." says Papa Bear. The three bears spoon some honey into Goldie Lock's mouth, and she soon revives. She sees the bears and runs away into the woods. THE END.

Everyone applauds. Very clever. And such great acting too. The next spot advertises an instant glucose mixture. All the kids exercise, doing jumping jacks. Soon they all fall down. Superman, or is it Sugarman, arrives on the scene. Peter, Sugarman, quickly pushes this magic formula into everyone's mouth, and they recover from their low blood sugar reactions. Moral of story: When exercising, always have an instant source of glucose with you. THE END.

Again we all clap. It is fun and educational. The next few acts need a little more polishing. But they, too, have potential. I love the one that takes place in the restaurant. Peter, Jeff, Becky, Susan, and Emily are seated around a table set with flowers and a bright tablecloth. (Emily points to herself on the TV screen.)

Susan, who has a big "D" on her forehead, brings out her blood glucose machine and proceeds to do a finger stick. Two of the diners, Becky and Emily, faint from the sight of blood, and fall to the floor. Then Susan takes out her syringe, draws up her insulin, and injects herself in the stomach. The other two, Peter and Jeff, dramatically fall on the floor. (I assume they have both watched many dying scenes on TV). The lone diner, Susan, awaits her meal. The waiter, Kevin, enters. "Your dinner, Madame." And she digs in for a good meal as the others remain on the floor. The screen goes blank.

This brings a hoot from the parents. Brent and Marjorie get into a laughing fit. Their daughter, not a natural ham, did a great job in the role of the compulsive, unfazed diabetic. These kids are clever.

"Bravo, Bravo!" Mark and Darryl shout. It is good to see them having fun. The kids want to rerun it once more. It is fun to see yourself on TV.

After the replay, Pat says, "Now, let's turn on the lights and sing just a few songs to prepare for Wednesday."

Some years we have singers and some years we don't. Pat and

I usually get up and clown around. This year Cindy and Nancy have lovely voices, but both are too shy and maybe too depressed to help us much tonight. Our last song of the night is "Little Bunny Phoo Phoo." This is Pat's yearly ritual. She is such a good sport and actress herself. She bounces around just as Little Bunny Phoo Phoo would and then plays a great good fairy.

We all applaud and laugh. "We'll do more singing on Wednesday at the campfire. Now, it's time for blood testing and snacks." Everyone moves out into the central hall.

I know now is the time. I work my way toward him. "Sam, can we talk?"

"Why not?" he replies.

"Let's go over to the French House where it will be quiet."

"Let me just go and kiss Emily good-night and tell my mom where we'll be."

He turns and walks up the stairs. He's so young, just 23. What a burden he's carrying. When I was 23, I had no children, no husband, and no diabetes. Just medical school. Well, I guess we all have some problems. The question is how do you work with those burdens and barriers. One of my patients once gave me a poster that said, "If Life Gives you Lemons, Make Lemonade." A rather flip answer for those with big lemons, like Sam's.

"Dr. MacCracken, do you want to play some ping-pong?" asks Kevin.

"Kev, it's almost 9 o'clock and time for quiet activities. I need to talk with Sam, but I promise I'll play. OK?"

"Sure. And this time you'd better play left-handed."

"It's a deal!" Kevin heads back into the playroom. Peter, Kyle, Jeff, and Susan are finishing a hockey foosball game, lots of rod twirling but few goals.

It's good to see Big Lucy talking with Lydia. I was concerned how Lydia would fit in. Her family is obviously the most indigent. But so far, she seems to be enjoying the activities, and mealtimes, too. All the adults are mixing well. All but Sam.

He comes back down the stairs with his red and black checked Maine jacket. His beard and his large size make him look a little older than 23. "I'm set," he says.

In silence we walk over to the French House. It's dark inside; no one is staying there. My heart is racing. I know how important it is to convince him to stay. I also know we can help him. But will the words be there when I need them? Will he even listen? I fumble for the light switch, which, I recall, is just inside the front door.

The chairs are all turned up on top of the tables. The floors have been swept. We pull two chairs down and sit. These chairs may not be too comfortable for long. Sam sits on his chair backwards, with his legs wrapped around and his arms draped over the back.

"My mom told you we're leaving in the morning?"

"Yes, she did. And I just wanted to find out why you need to go—and see if you'd be willing to listen to why I think you should stay."

There is a pause. He begins, "It was Mom and Ollie, my stepfather, wanted us to come here in the first place. Mom wants me to start taking care of Emily's diabetes. She's not sure she's doing it too good, and she says Emily needs me to take care of my diabetes, too. I'm sure you know I have diabetes."

"Yes, I do."

"Mom says Emily needs a good role model 'cuz she's growing up. And Mom doesn't think she got me the best care when I come down with diabetes, so she's hoping this camp would help that too. I'm sure my mom is right about a lot of this. But it isn't easy for me to admit I have diabetes to strangers. I figure it's my business, and I can handle it. Well, I was doing OK until . . . " His voice drifts off.

"Until, Rachel died." I had to say it.

"Yeah. She made me take care of myself. She wanted me to live for her."

"And Emily," I add. He is silent now. He looks away. I wonder if this is my chance. I stand by his chair and put my hand on his shoulder. He remains silent. His tears fall silently. He wipes them away with his sleeve and sniffs.

I pull some Kleenex out of my pocket. He takes it. "Sam, I'm very sorry about Rachel. Your mom told Pat and Pat told me. It must have been such a nightmare for you." He sniffs, and wipes. I think, God give me the words. "We all want you to stay. We'd really like to help you, and I think we can."

He keeps looking away, but the tears have turned into just heavy, long sighs. I move back to my chair.

"Your mother is right. Emily does need you. Besides your love, which I know you're giving her, she needs you to help her now with her diabetes. She needs to grow up thinking she and her daddy can take care of this. Right now I don't think she really knows what it's all about. Have you noticed that she only talks to you in whispers? Has everyone talked to you in whispers since your wife died?"

"No."

"Then, it is something that Emily has perceived. Maybe she's scared that you hate her diabetes and don't want to hear about it. It is hard for a five year old to separate herself from diabetes.

"Actually, it is hard for most people to keep those two things separate. She needs to meet other people, other kids with diabetes who are not afraid to say 'I have diabetes.' She needs to watch them do their blood tests without fear and take their injections without fuss.

"Five year olds do need examples, role models. We have some kids here like that. And she needs to have some fun. She needs to be able to let go of Pearl's hand and explore. Have you noticed? She is beginning to sit with Ginny and even participate in some games. She really laughed at the Bunny Phoo Phoo song."

Sam nods his head.

"And your mom. Sam, she needs this camp. She is trying so hard to do everything right. She is listening to every word of advice. I think she feels she failed you by not getting the best care for you in the beginning. She really didn't learn that much about your diabetes. Maybe you wanted to do it all on your own. At least she thinks she should have learned much more. And information changes, too. It's been seven years since you were diagnosed. Tests change, equipment changes. Your mom wants to do the best for Emily this time around."

"That's true."

"I know that if you stay, Emily will have a good time. She will blossom, surrounded with new special friends. She needs to laugh, and play again. And your mom will learn so much. She'll feel so much better about herself. She'll become more confident about the care she's giving Emily; I can promise you that. And what do I think we can offer you?" I'm quiet. Sam's quiet. Oh, please, words come now.

"Sam, let these folks become your friends. They've all felt the pain of diabetes. Eddy knows what it's like to be 16 or 17 with diabetes. Lucy and Lydia have had little ones with diabetes. They know the anguish of having to inject their own little child. These fathers know the feelings of being a dad with a child with diabetes.

"True, none of the parents here this year have diabetes, but we've had some parents with diabetes other years. One mother told us, it's harder being a parent of a diabetic child than having diabetes yourself. Both of you have the experience of seeing it both ways. Maybe you can be of some help to the folks here. Maybe you could give Brent or Darryl some help. Darryl is having a tough time with Becky. She hates her diabetes and is fighting it, too."

He's still listening.

"I wish I could have you talk to some of our past campers, especially two families who almost left but decided to stay. In the end they knew they had done the right thing. I'm sure we can help you get your diabetes under better control, if you want that. Nine years of experience at this camp has given me the confidence to say that sticking it out through the week will be worth it for Emily, Pearl, and you." Sam is quiet, looking down at the floor.

"Would you do me the favor and just sleep on it?" I ask.

"I'll think it over." We put our chairs back. As we leave, I turn out the light.

"Good night, Sam."

"Good night."

We walk away in different directions. He heads back to the main lodge. The flame of his cigarette lighter flickers in the darkness as he walks slowly back to the lodge. Turning towards our cabin, I see the lights are still on. Pat and Heather will be eager to hear how it went, and . . . I don't really know.

The sea mist has rolled in. There are no stars tonight.

Digging Deeper

Pat and Heather have already finished off most of the cheese and crackers. They're both knitting and talking about hospital matters.

"We thought we'd wait for you before we started discussing the campers," Pat comments.

"Any diet Coke left? I need something to drink after that conversation."

"Left-hand side of the fridge," says Pat. Before I come back into the living room to settle in for what could be a long talk, I put on my cozy sweater and some wool socks.

"Well, how do you want to do this? Should we go family by family and tell our initial impressions plus any important information we've learned?" Pat suggests.

"Sure, go for it. I'm a little tired from my talk with Sam, but I'll bounce back. Why don't you two start, and I'll add comments as we go along." The soda tastes good.

"Maybe, we should start with the easy ones first."

"Good idea."

Pat begins. "We all know Peter's family. I'm glad they came. Mark certainly is a great father and husband. I think he helps Lisa relax about Peter's diabetes. For awhile there she was pretty protective of him, but that's easing off. They have a good understanding of diabetes so far. Of course, he's still in the honeymoon phase, so his blood sugars are pretty easy to control on relatively small doses of insulin."

"He'll be coming out of that fairly soon. I've noticed on his chart that his blood sugars are running a little bit higher than they were when he was in clinic last month," I comment.

"Yeah, we'll have to watch that. Maybe we'll need to increase his insulin a bit," Pat says.

Heather says, "Abigail and Lucy are great little sisters. Abigail wants to be a nurse. Pat, she told me she wants to be just like you. That's a compliment. I was impressed with all the dietary information she knows too. Maybe she could do both of our jobs."

"The family seems to be pretty much together. I think Mark and Lisa took our suggestion at the time of Peter's diagnosis and have tried to spend time with Lucy and Abigail. Lisa coaches Abigail's soccer team, and Mark has a great relationship with little Lucy," Pat adds. "And boy, is Mark proud of Peter. He told me all about Peter's swimming at the YMCA and his soccer. Peter hasn't let his diabetes interfere with any of his sports. Eddy will be a great role model for him here."

"Let's just hope Peter stays as positive as he is now. It's still pretty new to him."

"Joan, don't be the doomsday predictor."

"I don't mean to be. I'm just being realistic. We all know that some of these well-controlled kids can become poorly controlled adolescents. It's a phase some have to go through during their separation from parental control."

"Speaking of phases, what about Becky's phase?" Heather comments.

"Yeah, that's some phase. You can't help noticing her negativism and the incredible way that she talks back to her mother. Everyone here has picked up on it, that's for sure," I add.

"Hard to miss it," says Heather.

Pat starts out. "I had a long talk with Nancy today, and she blames herself for it all. She's pretty discouraged. She knows she has a spoiled brat on her hands. She had two miscarriages before Becky, and ever since her birth, she's been spoiled. And then once the diabetes came along, it was even worse. Nancy has stayed home to care for Becky. In fact, Darryl is a salesman and travels a lot, and Nancy has had to make many decisions. But when it comes to discipline, she has always let Darryl take care of it. When he's away, Becky rules the roost."

"Darryl told me it's his fault," I interject. "He realizes that being away so much has been really hard on Nancy. He thinks she needs to get out of the house and start her singing career again. She was a very talented singer before they got married. Now his daughter is almost 13, and somehow he knows she needs to get more independent—and responsible."

"How are we going to help these folks? Becky really knows how to get to her mother and her dad. It's almost like they feel so guilty, they are helpless to do anything effective. But half the problem is solved, because both seem ready to change and both are aware that something must be done."

"I think Ginny will be able to help us some. She has such a good outlook on diabetes."

"And Cindy can help, too. Becky might just see that she's fairly lucky to have such loving and concerned parents compared with Cindy. She also might see that she is very fortunate to have so much. Did you see that stereo compact disc player in her room?"

"In addition to her Walkman."

"We've got some significant work to do with that family."

We all take a second to munch and sip. "Darn, I dropped a stitch. At this rate it will be Christmas before I'm done," Heather moans.

"I'm sure your dog won't mind if his Christmas present is late," I quip.

"Very funny, MacCracken," Heather retorts.

I continue. "Let me tell you one kid who is just great. That's Kyle. On the beach I asked him if Jeff got any special attention because of his diabetes. He just talked about how hard it was for his mom, and how his dad and he got to go bowling and ice fishing together. He and Jeff are really close. It's fun to see that in brothers. They're only a year apart."

51

"Jeff talks about Kyle too," Pat says. "He couldn't wait to tell Kyle about Goldie Locks and the Three Bears. Jeff was such a cute baby bear. And he's smart, too. He was the one who thought up the idea of Goldie Locks using his insulin all up. And then he knew she'd have a bad reaction. It was a great video session. All the kids enjoyed acting. It was fun, but Becky sure was bossy. Luckily, Ginny, as production manager, was able to control Becky's demands."

"Maybe Ginny needs to teach Darryl and Nancy. But I had something to say about Big Lucy," Heather adds. Oh, yes, she's limping more than I've seen her in the past. I bet her fingers are stiffer, too."

"It's hard for her to draw up Jeff's insulin, especially in the morning," Pat continues. "I'm going to work hard with Jeff this week to practice drawing it up just right. She'll still have to watch over him, but at least it won't be so painful for her. Steve's gone at such odd times with his new job. Jeff is going to have to learn himself. Steve feels bad about missing camp. But, obviously, he needs the job. I told him camp could help Jeff. I'll have extra time to spend with him. Lucy is a noble soul. I've never heard her complain."

"That's the truth." We all agree.

"Who's next?" I ask.

"Do you want to tell us about Sam? How did your talk go?"

"I really don't know. We had a good talk. I guess I did most of the talking. It was Pearl who made him come here. The hardest thing is facing the fact that Emily has diabetes. And, of course, he blames it all on himself. From father to daughter. And what a bummer that Rachel died. He might have slowly accepted Emily's diabetes with Rachel's love and help. But without it, he's just angry and depressed. I told him that Pearl needs this camp to learn more about diabetes to help Emily and that Emily needs to have some fun and learn to be less scared about leaving her grandmother. I told him I thought we could help him control his diabetes better if he is willing to try."

"So, what did he say?" asks Heather.

"Well, I asked him to sleep on his decision, and he said he

would. I have no clue if he'll decide to stay. But I sure hope he does."

"Well, you gave it your best, and we'll just have to see in the morning." Pat says.

"On that pleasant note should we move on to Lydia." We all look at each other. I actually haven't had too many words with Lydia except for supper on Sunday night. I've learned about her from Cindy, her daughter, but I'm eager to hear Pat and Heather's impression.

"Lydia knows lots about foods," says Heather. "When Brent asked how many fruit and fat exchanges there are in those new Flippits—those chocolate covered fruit snacks—Lydia said, 'Wait a minute, I'll go get a wrapper.' She went to her bedroom and came back with the box. So, you can see she has her own food stored upstairs."

"OK, what else have you learned about Lydia?"

"She makes and sells those figurines made out of lobster shells and claws."

"Really? You two ought to ask her to teach you how to do that. It could be your therapy project next year, Heather."

"Very funny, MacCracken."

"She must get her shells from her new boyfriend Lou," I comment.

Pat says, "Boy, did I get an earful about Lou from Kevin this afternoon. He hates Lou and says Lou is no good for his mother. Kevin likes being the only man in the house, or should I say mobile home."

"Did he tell you he has been in the hospital several times in the last few months."

"Well, he raised his hand when I asked the kids who had been in the hospital in the past six months. The only other kid who raised his hand was Peter, and that was when he was diagnosed in January. I didn't go into it during our group session with the other kids."

"Well, Cindy told me that Kevin's been skipping his insulin at times and wants to get into the hospital. He figures Lou won't want to be in a family with such a sick kid. Besides when he's in there, his mom and Lou don't get to be together as much."

Heather says. "Lydia told me she felt Kevin was overeating and getting himself sick. She has no idea that Kevin is skipping his shots. He's a sly fox."

"We need to talk with Kevin, obviously. But I don't have any idea how we can get him to accept Lou. Cindy says that her mom wants to get married, too. And Cindy doesn't see that as all bad either. She thinks her mom is happier around Lou. I think she's old enough to understand that her mom has been pretty lonely. I wish I could get Lydia to appreciate Cindy more. She really is a nice kid."

"Well, that's another family that needs some help."

"I'm fading fast, guys. How many families to go?"

"I think we've covered them all, except the Booths."

"I haven't had much contact with either of them yet. I sat with them at the first supper and later found out that Brent likes to play squash and that Marjorie is a librarian at Germantown Academy. But I haven't really gotten a strong feeling about them."

"Well, I have," Pat states.

"Me, too," says Heather. "You first."

"As far as I can tell this family gets the award for compulsive, uptight behavior. The only relaxed one is Tate. I'd guess Susan's diabetes is being controlled too tightly. She has had two reactions so far today, and we really haven't done any strenuous exercise. One reaction happened before lunch when they didn't let her have a mid-morning snack. The other, this afternoon came on for no apparent reason. I think she's on too much insulin."

"And they watch what she eats closely, too. They usually measure everything out at home on a scale. They're amazed we don't have a scale on each table in the dining hall. She gets precisely 1800 calories a day. That formula was calculated by Brent. He was taught that for each year of a child's life you add 100 calories to an already determined base calorie of 1,000."

"But she's ten and by that formula should be getting 2,000 calories."

"Correct, Dr. MacCracken," Heather smiles, "but he has decided his daughter's an inactive child. Because she sits and reads all the time, he's deducted 200."

"Maybe, for activity, he should add calories onto that formula instead of deducting for inactivity," I comment.

"In addition, both Brent, who, by the way, is a mathematician at the University of Pennsylvania, and his wife have been taught to use an incredibly tight range for Susan's blood sugars. They are aiming for 70 to 120, and when they check her two hours after the meals and find her higher than that, they increase her dose."

"Ouch! That's certainly going to lead to problems."

"I think it already has. She must be having reactions all the time. I really don't think she looks very healthy, do you?"

"No, I noticed her rather pasty complexion and chipmunk face. She may be putting out a lot of *counterregulatory hormones* in response to those reactions. I need to talk to them about *rebound* and the problems of *hypoglycemia*."

"That might not be too easy. Brent has a lot of faith in their doctor who set those glucose ranges."

"Sounds more like an adult diabetologist who deals with pregnant women with diabetes. They do have to control their blood sugars much more tightly for the health of the baby. I suppose they could have misinterpreted his instructions. We all know that can happen."

"I think Brent said her doctor was an internist. She's never been to the Children's Hospital."

"How much insulin is she on?

"I think she is taking quite a bit over one unit per kilogram, but I haven't weighed her. Marjorie said she was 95 pounds, which is heavy for a 10-year-old, isn't it? She also said Susan is having trouble keeping her weight down."

"It is probably all that excess insulin causing fat to be laid down. I bet we could help her hold her weight down by decreasing her insulin some. "

"I bet she'd feel better, too. She probably doesn't know what feeling good is like," Heather adds.

Pat continues. "Have you seen her record book? She uses five different colors to chart, depending on the value. I think they give her extra regular, too, if she gets above 180. They have a "sliding scale" for determining the extra insulin requirement. Brent told me their doctor suggested the scale."

"I'm not sure that doctor and I would see eye to eye. I'll just have to give the Booths my reasoning for our insulin recommendations and see if I can make it make sense to them. They certainly are smart enough. Maybe they haven't been given enough information to make their decisions."

"Sounds like another little project for this week."

"We better get to bed. I wanted to talk about Ginny and Eddy, but they seem to be doing OK. Don't you think?

"I think we chose two great counselors this year."

"Well, tomorrow is our big day. Do you think the troops are ready?"

"I guess so. They all seem to know each other now. I hope Sam, Pearl, and Emily will be with us. Most of this group seems to be in touch with their feelings. I'm not sure about Brent and Marjorie. They may be pretty guarded. We'll see. Be sure to bring the Kleenex box. What time is Tim arriving?"

"He said he'd try to be here for breakfast. He was really sorry he couldn't come tonight. You know how he likes to have time with the campers before he has to run the group session. We'll just have to fill him in fast."

"He is so good—and sensitive I'm sure everything will be fine."

"Well, this has been one very busy day. I have a feeling it's going to be a good week," Pat says.

By this time, Heather is about asleep on the couch. We turn off the lights and suggest she climb into her bed.

"You guys probably expect me to get up at the crack of dawn, too. I tell you I need my beauty rest."

"Good night, Heather." We all head to our beds. It's been just over 24 hours of camp, and we all know we have several challenges to tackle in the next five days.

Looking Back,
Thinking Ahead

"Oh, the Lord is good to me,
And so I thank the Lord
For giving me the things I need,
The sun and the rain and the insulin,
The Lord is good to me."

Not a bad rendition for breakfast grace, especially on such a foggy morning. I hear Nancy's and Cindy's beautiful voices, one a strong soprano and the other a rich alto.

Tim Rogers walks in as we are just digging into our hot cereal and freshly made banana bread. The dark circles under his eyes hint that his job as Director of the Behavioral and Developmental Department at the hospital may be taking its toll. One year he stayed here for the entire week, and I think he enjoyed the change. But he can't afford the time away from the hospital and must settle for one day here. Maybe someday when he gets more help, he'll be able to stay longer. I'm just glad he's here today to help with our designated "feelings day." After my talk with Sam last night I could use some reinforcements.

I look over at Sam, who has said nothing to me this morning. Pearl, Emily, and Sam were late for the breakfast bell. I assume they were packing. Maybe after breakfast he'll at least tell me his decision. His slight smile at Pat confuses me.

Pat announces, "We'll meet at 9 o'clock for our morning session. This afternoon is our mud hike. Tim, our bearer of good news, says that it is sunny in Bangor and predicts the fog will clear before lunch. And if it's warm enough, maybe we can try the water slide."

"All right!" shouts Jeff, our go-getter. He's been checking out the hill's slope ever since he arrived. The plastic water slide is one of the most exciting activities for the kids here. Jeff had a great time on the water slide when he was here two years ago at the grandparent-grandchild camp. He can't wait to show his brother Kyle how fast he can go. Guaranteed, he'll be first in line.

"Dishes this morning are Sam, Mark, and Peter, a totally male crew. Can you handle it, men?" Pat jokes.

"In no time," Mark comments, rising to the occasion. The other campers head for the door. Heather, Pat, Tim, and I pour ourselves another round of coffee. We need to discuss the morning session and fill Tim in on our observations.

Pearl and Emily leave. As Sam walks toward the kitchen, he stops by my chair, bends over, and whispers in my ear.

"We've decided to stay. And thanks for last night." He heads over to join the all-male dishwashing team.

"Here comes our dryer," Mark says to Peter, as Sam enters the kitchen. Pat and Heather see my smile and instantly know there will be no one leaving today.

Tim is quick to pick up on some of the personalities. Somehow he has already noted Brent's and Marjorie's controlling ways. They were sitting next to him at breakfast. We warn him of Sam's precarious emotional state, of Darryl and Nancy's despair, of Cindy's longings and Kevin's jealousies and manipulations. At 9 we head over for the morning session. Tim's sensitivity and experience will have to take care of the rest.

In the meeting room everyone finds a seat in the big circle. I begin.

"This morning we are fortunate to have with us Dr. Tim Rogers from Eastern Maine Medical Center. He's a pediatric psychologist and has worked with Pat, Heather, and me for several years. Tim always comes on the day we have a mud hike because he loves to get his sneakers muddy. I'll let him tell you what he has planned for us."

Tim is dressed in dark green shorts and a yellow T-shirt. His casual manner puts people at ease. "I'm always happy to come down to Hersey Retreat. It's true I love the mud hike. But this morning we're going to try and deal with feelings. You all know that there are no right and wrong feelings—just feelings, strong ones, not so strong ones. We can feel happy, sad, frustrated, angry, nervous, shy, upset, peaceful, quiet, friendly, embarrassed, et cetera. Today maybe we can help identify some of our feelings." The group is quiet.

He continues, "For my sake, would you just go around and state your name, so I can begin to get to know you. If you give me last names, I'll be able to put the families together." Fairly quickly the campers go around and say their names. Tim mentally registers the faces with the names of the people we talked about at breakfast.

"Thanks. Now to start with, we're going to act out some skits, just brief ones. For the first one I need volunteers to play a mother, a father, and a doctor." No one immediately volunteers. I hate to role play and understand everyone's hesitation. Tim usually waits for volunteers. Occasionally as the session progresses, he will call on selected individuals if he thinks it may be therapeutic. Pat volunteers to be the mother, Mark McCabe volunteers to be the father, and Tim suggests to Eddy that he play the doctor. Eddy gets a kick out of this. He once considered being a doctor. But now he wants to be a teacher.

Tim's index cards tell the actors and actresses what they are to do. He tells the campers to determine what is going on in the skit and put that into words. Pat and Mark sit facing Eddy, who has taken on a rather pretentious air as the doctor.

"Mr. and Mrs. Jones, your child, Junior, has Type I insulin-dependent diabetes mellitus."

"Diabetes, no. That can't be, there's no diabetes in our family," the mother comments.

"How long has he had it? I just can't believe it?" questions the father.

"Junior has only exhibited the symptoms of *polyuria, polydipsia*, and weight loss for about two weeks, but his pancreas has been under attack by his autoimmune system for quite some time."

"You mean his drinking and urinating a lot were late signs?"

"Will he get over it when his immune system stops attacking?"

"How long will we have to treat him?"

"I'll try to answer your questions. There need not be any diabetes in the family history. It is not entirely controlled by the genes and the *HLA system*." Eddy laughs, being impressed with his up-to-date medical vocabulary. Pat is impressed with Eddy, too. "He will require insulin for the rest of his life. His pancreas no longer produces sufficient amounts of insulin. Thus, to control the hyperglycemia, the high blood sugar, he must receive insulin by subcutaneous injection."

"You mean shots? Oh, I just can't believe it!"

"This is such a shock!" Pat and Mark comfort each other.

"You'll have to excuse me. I need to see my other patients. The nurse educator will be in to see you this afternoon."

Pat, Mark, and Eddy look up as though they are finished. I notice that Nancy has been wiping tears away discretely.

"Does anyone want to tell what these actors were doing?"

"It's the first time the parents have heard the diagnosis," comments Big Lucy.

"Right," says Tim. "Anything else?"

"The parents don't want to believe it," Kevin adds.

"Good point, anything else?"

"The doctor is using big words like they do," says Kevin.

"You got it," says Eddy. "I was supposed to act aloof and

scientific with little feeling."

"That was well done," Tim says. He looks over in Nancy's direction. She wipes her eyes again. Tim takes one step towards Nancy and with a very gentle voice states, "That was difficult for you, Nancy." She nods her head. Everyone else is quiet.

"I thought I had finished crying over this. But it was such a hard time for me. I cried and cried for weeks. Becky is my only child, and I had such a hard time having her that I guess I had expected everything to be perfect for her." She reaches out for the Kleenex from Pat.

Her husband Darryl adds, "And our doctor wasn't very understanding. He acted so matter of fact about it. To us it was like dropping the atom bomb on us." Becky listens.

"I agree," says Lydia, who also reaches for some tissue. "It was such a shock. Kevin was pretty sick when we got him to the hospital. He had been getting skinnier, but I didn't know why. He was eating a lot and peeing a lot, too. I never heard of those things related to diabetes. My sister-in-law with diabetes is overweight, not skinny. The doctor said we brought Kevin in just in time. He was almost in a coma." She wipes her eyes again.

"It's very scary when you learn that your child has diabetes," I say. Most everyone nods their heads. The kids are quiet. Becky and Kevin watch their mothers weep. Cindy watches her mom, too.

"I was scared when Mommy and Daddy left Peter at the hospital," says Abigail. "I was afraid he wouldn't come back. They tried to tell me and my sister about diabetes, but we were so scared about the shots. I remember I cried that night." Her mother grabs Abigail's hand and squeezes her daughter, Lucy, who is sitting on her lap. Mark, the actor father and real father, looks over at Peter.

These are the important moments, as this sharing begins. Tim, Pat, Heather, and I all keep our eyes out for the hurting soul who may need our loving attention.

"Here's another skit that isn't so hard. I need a father, a mother, and two kids."

Peter and Jeff raise their hands, stand up simultaneously, and walk over to Tim. Pearl volunteers for the mother and Darryl, the father. Tim shows them the index card, and they have a small conference together.

Darryl and Pearl sit in two seats, and the two boys sit in two seats behind their actor parents. From experience I know this is an automobile. Darryl starts to drive with his hands around an imaginary wheel and to talk about the traffic. Jeff says, "How much longer 'til we get there? I'm hungry."

"We should be there in about half an hour. Why don't you take your shot now, and then you'll be ready to eat when we get to Grandma's," says the mother.

"She usually has supper waiting for us," comments the father.

Jeff and Peter start to look for things in the back of the car. Jeff's face takes on a small panicky expression. "Mom, I can't find my insulin bag. Didn't you pack it?"

"No, I thought you put it in your backpack."

Jeff replies, "I left it on the counter in the kitchen. Oh no, what are we going to do without my insulin and syringes."

"Well, we'll just have to get to Grandma's house and call the pharmacy and maybe Dr. MacCracken," says Darryl.

The car driving comes to an end. The participants look around having nothing more to say. Tim asks for comments.

"That happened to us too when we were driving to my grammy's," comments Tate. "I got carsick, too." His mother frowns.

Susan, who has been very quiet, quickly adds, "My father had an extra prescription for syringes. He always makes sure to carry one. And we had some insulin at my grandmother's house in the refrigerator. Without that, we would have been stuck."

Brent, Susan's dad, adds, "These predicaments certainly do arise. I've found it's good to plan ahead. We try to carry extra insulin bottles in case one breaks." Folks nod their heads, as though they've all broken a bottle or two. "Our doctor told us to always carry an extra prescription for syringes because in this age of drugs, syringes can be very hard to obtain even in an emergency."

"Good point, Brent," I comment. I don't want this to get off the track of feelings. We could easily drift into the subject of equipment supply problems, but not today. That's for Thursday. "How have others reacted to these problems?"

"They just don't understand," says Kevin. He stops.

"Kevin, what do you mean?" asks Tim.

"Well, once I had a teacher take away my syringe from my bag. He thought I was into drugs or something. He didn't know I had diabetes, and when I tried to tell him, he didn't believe me."

"Kev, that teacher is about the dumbest guy in our school," adds his sister Cindy, sympathetically.

"Yeah, well, the principal made him apologize to me after."

"How did that make you feel?"

"It made me mad that he didn't believe me at first, but it was great that he had to apologize. I guess he had to learn a little about diabetes, too. The principal gave him a book on diabetes for teachers. He's pretty nice to me now. But there are still some jerky kids who don't have no clue about diabetes. You wouldn't believe what some think." Kevin shakes his head.

Becky speaks up. "One girl in my school thinks she can catch it from me. I sometimes threaten I'll give it to her if she won't let me cut in line for lunch.

"Becky, that's terrible," says her father.

"Becky's angry at the ignorance of this girl. But maybe it would be better though if Becky did a science project on diabetes and tried to teach her class about it," Pat says. Becky appears to think about that, but just shrugs.

Then she adds, "I don't really care. It's none of their business, anyway."

"Pat came to my school and gave a puppet show for my class. It was great. They learned about diabetes and even wanted to see my blood testing machine and see me give my own injection," comments Peter enthusiastically.

For many years Pat has been visiting schools in our region after a child with diabetes is diagnosed. Her office walls are covered with thank-you notes from the classes, who genuinely enjoy learning about diabetes. I think it takes the fear away, fearful thoughts like, "Can I catch it? Will I get it from eating too many candy bars? Can I catch it from my cat?" Pat marvels at some of their concerns. Many kids in our clinic have done detailed science projects on diabetes. It gives them a better handle on the disease, as a separate entity from themselves.

Tim says, "Let's try another skit. For this one I need someone to play a teenage brother of a sister with diabetes and someone to play his mother. Do I have any volunteers?

After the last skit most everyone understands the idea, but still no one eagerly volunteers. Ginny agrees to play the mother, a role she has not yet experienced. Tim says he loves to play teenage boys, so he'll give this one a try.

Ginny looks at the index card. Tim already knows his role. They sit down opposite each other.

"Tim, will you do the dishes tonight, please?"

"It isn't my turn, it's Shelley's."

"Shelley has to get her homework done tonight because she has her diabetes clinic tomorrow morning."

"So what! I had soccer practice, and I have lots to do, too."

"Tim, do the dishes!"

"It's just not fair. You're always giving her special privileges, and she never has to do all the chores I do. Just because she has diabetes doesn't mean she shouldn't have to do chores."

"Tim, you are being unreasonable. I just asked you to do the dishes."

"You spend so much more time with her, too, and all we get to eat around here is rabbit food—carrots, celery, and rice cakes. Why do I have to eat what she eats? All my friends think I'm weird with those rice cakes. Where are the cookies we used to have?" Tim is hitting some important points.

"Tim, you know it takes time to work with Shelley, and we have discussed our approach to her diet before. What has gotten into you?"

They both look up and stop there. Looking around the room there are some smiling folks who are impressed with Tim's and Ginny's acting, but Lydia and Cindy are both weeping. And Marjorie is blotting her eyes. Tim switches character and tone of voice and directs his question to Marjorie. "That one must have hit a tender spot?"

Marjorie straightens up a bit, possibly not wanting Tate to notice her sadness. She begins to speak, but the words are hard to find. She tries again. "With four kids it's hard to spread my time evenly. I work as a librarian, and Brent is busy with his courses. I'm afraid that Tate is getting only the time left over. After four kids, and with the third having the diabetes, I guess Tate has had to fend for himself a lot." She looks over at her son.

"Mom, I'm tough," Tate scoffs as he flexes his muscle. Everyone laughs. Tate's a perceptive six-year-old. This light interjection briefly allows the group to relax, but only momentarily. There's more work to be done.

"Lydia, you took that one hard, too." comments Tim. "And Cindy."

Pat and I look at each other. This might be a tough part coming up. But this is the time, and it's the right environment. Many parents here have felt guilty about giving more time to the child with diabetes. Some parents are able to juggle their children's needs better. If both Lydia and Cindy can express their feelings, maybe they'll feel better about each other. Kevin watches both.

I look at my watch. It's almost time for snack, but this would not be a good time to interrupt. Usually we break and then go on with only the older kids and parents. Now, we continue.

"What was so hard for you, Lydia?"

"It just hurts," she sighs. No one speaks. "I guess I haven't done a very good job. Being mom and dad to these two kids is tough, and the diabetes makes it tougher." She wipes her tears. "Kevin's always in the hospital, and I worry about Cindy being home alone. I mean she is 13 now, and I don't think she's got the best kind of friends."

"Mom, I told you," Cindy interrupts.

Tim stops her. "Cindy, wait. Let your mother finish."

Lydia takes another deep breath. "Our case worker thinks I don't take care of Kevin—that I'm not a good enough mom to keep him. She thinks his going into the hospital all the time is my fault. But, I swear, I try to watch what he eats and make sure he has his insulin. But Kevin is 11 now, and he's smart enough to do whatever he pleases. I'm not going to let them take him away from me."

Her pitch increases. She's almost yelling and is on the edge of her seat. "I just don't think it's all my fault." She sits back in her chair.

The group is silent. Everyone feels her pain, her anger, her despair, and her desperation. Nancy and Marjorie have been wiping their tears throughout this session. Sam, who has been standing up behind his mother, has his hand on her shoulder. Pearl reaches up and holds on to her son's hand. They have all felt and feel the pain.

"Let's take a ten minute break and then come back here to share some more," I say. The rather rapid movement of chairs confirms my impression. We all need a break. The group files out into the hall where the snacks are. Kevin, Cindy, and Lydia stay.

Tim speaks to them, as Pat and I stand by. "You all need to keep talking. It's hard, I know, but these are important things to get out, and with these supportive people around, this is a good time."

Kevin looks at his mom. I wonder if he'll be willing to admit to his manipulative behavior and to reveal his reasons. I doubt all of this will come out. Others in the group need to vent. Though we direct the conversation slightly during these sessions, most campers volunteer their comments. When one starts opening up, others follow with candor.

Out in the hall, the kids surround the snack table as if they all need food. Even the adults take a cracker or two. Snack time for the children with diabetes is a fairly traditional way of dividing up calories. Most children are initially put on three meals a day and a mid-morning, mid-afternoon and bedtime snack.

Snack times should occur when insulins have their maximum effect and should ideally provide enough calories to keep the child from having low blood sugar before the next meal. The timing of insulin and meals is a very important part of diabetes management. At camp we try to show flexibility is still possible for snacks and mealtimes.

This snack break is about twenty minutes late, and yet no one appears to be having any problem. In fact many older children and adults with diabetes don't even take a mid-morning snack. Our society has almost always planned mid-morning snacks for the smaller children. It's part of nursery school and grammar school, at least in the lower grades.

In high school not only are snack times not scheduled, but lunches occur anytime from 11 to 1 and may last only 17 minutes. I recall one teenager in our clinic who had to juggle having lunch at different times each school day. That's a real challenge.

The adults surround the coffee urn. Perhaps, everyone needs a morning pick-me-up. The fog has not lifted yet, though it feels a bit warmer. I sure hope Tim's right about that sunshine. We'll need some cheery weather after this heavy morning.

Heather heads upstairs to the third floor with Little Lucy, Emily, Jeff, Kyle, Tate, and Susan. I'm sure Heather would prefer to stay with the adult group, but for years Pat has taken the kids, and she expressed a desire to stay for the second half of the morning. Heather makes great T-shirt designs, so even though six children at once may not be exactly her cup of tea, I know they'll have fun.

Eddy and Ginny, our counselors, want to stay with the parents. Pat and I are pleased. Both have lived with diabetes, and these parents will listen carefully to their words. Pat, Tim, and I have only learned from others. Of course, Sam has had those experiences too, but I'm not sure he will share them, yet.

Back in the meeting room we pull the chairs into a smaller circle. The youngest child in the room is Abigail, nurse-to-be. She's a concerned sister. If she carries this sensitivity into her adulthood, she'll make a fantastic nurse. She sits between Pat and her brother, Peter. Mark and Lisa must have told Peter and Abigail they could stay. If they felt it necessary to shield them from these discussions, they could have sent them upstairs. I hope it will be okay. The only other young campers are Kevin, Cindy, and Becky. Becky didn't say much in the morning session, but I hope she was listening. It's painful for any child to see his or her mother cry. Her external veneer of hostility (mainly directed at her mother) and self-centeredness appear thick, but surely she could feel her mother's pain.

Ginny and Eddy sit next to each other. They look so eager to help. And Sam and Pearl sit right next to me. I can sense a closeness with Sam. I only wish he would share some of his pain, or even just be able to say he has diabetes. I'm sure some of the parents know, but Sam has got to be able to say it and then go on.

During the break, Tim said he wants to cover several different topics and get some others to participate. Actually, the group looks eager to continue sharing. Probably this is the first time many of them have had this many people around with similar concerns. The relaxed and friendly environment encourages the flood gates to open and release those disturbing and frustrating feelings.

"We've talked about the pain of diagnosis, the frustrations of the daily routine, shots, extra insulin, the anger and jealousy of siblings, and the difficulty in balancing family times. What other feelings have you had to confront?" Tim says.

Pearl opens up. "Somebody commented on the stupidity of others or maybe, I guess Pat said it, the fear of others. What hurts me is when Emily isn't invited to any little birthday parties. She doesn't understand it. Many of Emily's friends can't have Emily over to play unless I go with her. I guess the mothers are afraid something might happen to Emily, and they won't know what to do."

"We initially had that problem, too," comments Lucy. "Jeff was very upset with his T-ball coach, who made him sit out a lot and was afraid to let him play too hard. Jeff's father and I talked with the coach. Several years before, one of the little players with diabetes had a bad low blood sugar reaction in the outfield, and that scared the coach. I explained to him about food and exercise and promised to always have Jeff well-fed before practice or a game. That helped.

"People who are not around people with diabetes all the time are afraid of it. We just need to explain things to them. My own mother was afraid to have Jeffrey spend the afternoon alone with her. Both of my boys love to go to their grandmother's house, but she just felt too nervous with Jeff's diabetes. The best thing we ever did was to have her come to Camp Grand with Jeffrey. She learned so much and gained confidence in caring for him. Pearl, as a grandmother, you are doing a remarkable job."

"Thank you. I've had to learn to."

Darryl speaks. "This might go along with what Nancy already said, but I have had to try to accept the fact that Becky is physically disabled. She just doesn't seem to be able to keep up with the other kids. And you look ahead and think about the problems that diabetics can have like . . . , well, you know, with their eyes and kidneys and legs."

I know he means blindness, kidney failure, and amputations. He continues, "I guess when I drive away on a sales trip, I try to put all of that out of my mind. Then I don't have to deal with it, but I feel bad, because I know that I'm leaving Nancy home to handle it."

Ginny speaks. "You can't pity Becky. That's not what those of us with diabetes need or want. You have to believe that the fact we have diabetes is just . . . well, just an annoyance. Sure, we have to take shots twice or three times a day. We can get used to that. And sure we'd all like to have more freedom to eat whatever we want, but the basic fact is that we happen to have diabetes. I, for one, refuse to consider myself disabled. In fact I despise that word.

"No one with diabetes is disabled unless complications set in. And there are plenty of people with diabetes who have not had their limbs cut off or lost their vision or kidneys. We have to believe we can do anything in life that anyone else can do, as long as we eat well and take our insulin."

Wow, that's quite a statement! Ginny has her uncle to thank for that attitude. And she, like him, is going to make a powerful lawyer who just happens to have diabetes. I'd hate to be the opposing lawyer. She's one determined young woman.

I look at Peter and Abigail. This is all new to them. Peter has only had diabetes six months. I hope it isn't too hard on him to hear about the amputations . Maybe he hasn't heard of that part yet. On Thursday he'll hear about the great and encouraging therapies for prevention of blindness in diabetes, but talk of amputations is probably very frightening for him and his parents. It's frightening for any of us. It's not something we usually discuss at this age. Mark leans over and whispers something in Peter's ear. Peter nods as though he understands his father's comment. Then Abigail hears the same message from her dad.

"I agree with Ginny," Eddy adds. "I'm in great shape. I work at it, that's true." That is true, he has a body like an Olympic athlete. "And no one in my class thinks of me as disabled. Some of them joke that my insulin injections must be power medicine when they clock my time running the bases. There are many great athletes with diabetes who play professional sports. Diabetes hasn't stopped them. And many famous movie stars, like Mary Tyler Moore, have diabetes. They just fit their diabetes management into their busy work schedules.

"I'm sure you have to learn to be flexible in your scheduling, but it can be done. Dr. MacCracken helped me figure out a special insulin program when I had to play double headers. I think it's the people without the diabetes that have more problems accepting us as normal. They're the ones who get freaked by the shots and blood tests. If we act like it's no big deal, then maybe they'll learn, too."

Score two for the counselors. I think this is all unrehearsed, though I'm sure that both Eddy and Ginny have been vocal about their diabetes in their schools. Ginny is class president this year and aiming for Harvard. And Eddy made the All-State Baseball Team. I think he said he holds the state stolen base record. Mark whispers something else in Peter's ear. I'll bet he knows Eddy's batting average.

Big Lucy has been listening intently. No, she would never want to be called disabled either. She may limp some, and her fingers may be quite stiff, so maybe that's reason enough for the label. She comments, "I think Eddy and Ginny have great attitudes, and though each of them may go through some ups and downs, I just want to encourage them to keep striving for all they can do. Those who give in to their difficulties will only start a vicious cycle of defeatism. One day Jeff came home from school and said, 'I'm glad I'm a diabetic and not a vegetarian. The kid who sits next to me is a vegetarian, and he can't have pepperoni pizza. Poor kid.' I guess it's all the way we look at things."

"Well, I don't want diabetes, and I hate all this stuff we're supposed to do," Becky shouts. "It's easy for parents to say 'do this' and 'do that,' but you don't have diabetes. It's a lot easier for you. You're not the one taking the shots."

Becky is an angry young lady. It isn't hard to understand her parents' desperation. But, she's up front about it, and that's a positive sign. Kevin is all ears. Perhaps Becky is vocalizing some of his inner most feelings. The whole group is quiet. No one wants to have diabetes. No one wants anyone else to have it, either. We all want to find a cure. Doctors, nurses, dietitians, parents. We all wish it would go away.

"Becky, you sound so much like I did when I got diabetes." There, he said it. All eyes are on Sam. From their expressions I can tell few knew he had diabetes.

"I didn't want diabetes, I still don't want it," he continued." That feeling hasn't changed. But what I think you need to know is that it hurts even more to have your own child get diabetes.

"When the doctor said Emily had diabetes, I just wouldn't believe it. And worrying about her and trying to do what is best for her and trying to keep her healthy and trying to control her glucoses so she'll stay well is a major job, a burden, a gigantic responsibility. And . . . ," he is almost weeping. "It's been so tough to face. I guess I've just about given up trying." He buries his head in his hands. I put my hand on his back. Pearl puts her hand on his thigh. No one speaks for a moment.

"It's true, Becky. Your mother and I would both take on diabetes if it would take it from you. I'm sure every parent in this room would give up all they have to rid their child of diabetes. Sam knows our pain and yours ."

Becky's father looks lovingly at her. Her mother wipes her tears, and her body language expresses her motherly desire to give Becky a big hug. Becky looks away and down, maybe as though she might regret some of her hostility.

Tim looks over at me. Is there more to cover? Have these folks felt enough today? Has the sharing made them feel any better? Hard to tell. But as long as it keeps rolling on its own, let's not stop now.

Eddy starts to speak. "I can understand what Sam is saying, because my little sister just came down with diabetes. She and Peter were in the hospital the same week. It bothers me more to know she has diabetes than it does that I have it. I guess that sounds strange, but it's true. I guess I feel like I can take care of myself, but I'm concerned about her. I can just imagine how my parents feel now that they have two kids to worry about."

"Does that happen very often, Dr. MacCracken? I mean having two kids in one family get diabetes? What are the statistics on that?" Brent, the mathematician, asks.

"The overall chance of having another child come down with diabetes is about 5%. You can find out a more accurate risk prediction by doing genetic studies on the child with diabetes and the siblings. Those who have a certain area of the chromosome very similar or identical to the child with diabetes will have a higher risk. If the gene area, what we call the HLA type, is completely different than the child with diabetes, then that sibling is very unlikely to develop diabetes.

"It's interesting that even if the HLA types are identical, as in identical twins, the risk is only 40 to 50% that both twins will get diabetes. That implies there are other factors besides just genetics. Eddy and his sister are only the second set of siblings we follow in our clinic of about 150 patients. We also had one other family here at camp with two sisters with diabetes. Only about 15% of new cases have any first-degree relatives—parents or siblings—with diabetes. So it really is not that common."

"I read an article in *Diabetes Forecast* once where there were four or maybe it was five kids with diabetes in one family," said Nancy.

"Oh, God, just think of all the supplies," comments Brent.

We are drifting away from the emotional realm, but maybe everyone has had enough for today. The smallest patch of blue sky is visible off in the distance. It just may clear.

"I'd like to say one more thing," Ginny requests. "Darryl was talking about disabilities and what diabetics can't do. It seems to me that those of us with diabetes could use our diabetes to our selfish advantage if we want to. All of us with diabetes know that you can manipulate your environment. If you wanted to, you could be sick all the time, eat too much, not check your bloods, forget your shots, and ignore things. That could certainly get you some attention. And you could use it to call attention to yourself in school too—like make a big deal about your blood testing or your snacks.

"I remember at cheerleading camp this one girl who made such a big deal about her diabetes. I think she wanted to get the coach to pity her. I suppose diabetes could be used as a crutch or even as a weapon. I just know I don't want to be known as a diabetic—and a weak one at that.

"Sure, I think for safety others should know you have diabetes, just in case you have a reaction or something, but otherwise, I want to be treated just like the next person."

Ginny looks around, and Big Lucy gives her a warm smile. Kevin looks glum. Did that hit home. Boy, it's almost like I told Ginny to say that. But, I haven't discussed Kevin's situation with her. And I'm quite sure that Pat and Heather haven't either. Then, I spot Cindy. She looks pleased. Maybe Cindy and Ginny have been doing some talking. It wouldn't surprise me if Ginny decided to try to convince Kevin that his manipulative ways are unfair and dangerous.

"Does anyone have anything else to say?" Tim asks.

We all look around the room. We've covered a lot, many thoughts to ponder, an emotional roller coaster ride. Little Lucy comes flying through the swing doors, "Look at my T-shirt, Mommy." Tate and Emily arrive next, wearing their newly designed shirts. Emily has a big flower on the front with a little rabbit sitting underneath. I bet Heather helped her make that one.

"See my bunny. Heather put it under the flower." Pearl gives her granddaughter a big hug and kiss. Emily is a beautiful little girl.

Tim quickly draws the session to a close. He encourages the everyone to keep sharing with each other throughout the week.

As the sun breaks through, Pat and I go outside to watch the final patches of fog clear off the bay. With the tide out, seal rock is visible. In fact I think I can even see Old Mr. Seal, sitting there just waiting for the sun's full warmth.

"That was quite a morning," Pat says. "Certainly used up our supply of Kleenex."

"I'd say so," I add. "I was really glad that Sam spoke up. I think he's going to be OK."

Pat nods. "This should be a fun afternoon. Did you remember your old sneakers?" She gives me a punch in the arm. She knows me so well. There are times I'd misplace my head, if it weren't attached.

CHAPTER 6

Reacting to Reactions

We have a brief rest hour. We all could use a longer quiet time, but the tide is coming in, and if we wait too long, we won't be able to get back across the stream without swimming. The sun is pouring down its warmth now. A warm, blue sky day in Maine, with a gentle, cool sea breeze can't be beat in my book. And it looks like the Philadelphia and Ohio families think so, too.

Everyone is ready for the hike. Even Big Lucy has her old sneakers on. Marjorie is wearing sandals. That won't do, so I loan her an old pair of sneakers. All the kids are eager to get going. Eddy's flashy hot pink trunks and his black fluorescent Boston Hard Rock Cafe tank top are "awesome." Kevin has on some tattered jeans. He tells me he never wears shorts. Lydia whispers that she'd rather not go. Beach hikes are not her thing. And, besides, she doesn't have anything, but flipflops. I realize it might be a tough walk for her, because of her excessive weight. Nancy has a headache and prefers to stay out of the bright sun. Those are the only two staying behind. Perhaps, they'll have some quiet time to share.

Pat calls everyone. "Gather round. We're going to walk down to the beach, along the mudflats, which are probably a little under water, an inch or two. If it's warm enough, Eddy might even go in for a dip. Some of you with bathing suits on might get a chance to get wet. Don't go out any further than Eddy, though. Actually, with the mud flats it won't get too deep," Pat adds.

"Be sure to tie your shoes on tight. Sometimes they get stuck in the mud," I add. "You should use some sunscreen, too. We don't want any sunburns tonight." Marjorie rubs some lotion on Tate's nose. Susan waits in line for sunscreen for her exposed shoulders.

Pat and Tim bring juice, oranges, raisins, crackers, and cheese in their backpacks.

"Dr. MacCracken, do you have any buckets?" asks Abigail.

"Good idea, Abigail. In the treasure chest." She and Little Lucy go to the chest and get three plastic buckets. Abigail hands one to Emily, who is delighted.

I'm pleased to see Sam interacting with the other fathers. I bet they have many questions for him now that they know he has diabetes, too. The mud hike provides the perfect setting for the adults to talk as their children splash and explore the beach front.

"If everyone is ready, let's go!" Pat grabs Emily and Little Lucy's hands, and the three skip down the grassy path, buckets flying.

Eddy, Ginny, and the rest of the kids except Susan run after them, and we follow behind. Susan takes my hand and walks quietly along. I'm still worried about her insulin dosage and haven't talked to her parents about lowering it yet. I plan to. They seem so determined that she must never have a high blood sugar.

Tim Rogers and Cindy stroll down the path, too. He and Cindy sat together at lunch and then spent the rest hour talking. I'm sure Tim can give Cindy some good counseling. She needs to feel better about herself. And somehow, her mother Lydia has got to see Cindy's strong points.

Passing down the open grassy field and into the woods the group hikes. Everyone chatters about this and that. Some campers haven't been down to the beach yet. The seagulls are flying all around. As the wooded path opens to the beach, we can see the clammers digging on the flats. The gulls love to hover, hoping for handouts. Three men are bent over filling their wooden baskets with mussels and clams. Their rakes move rapidly.

"What are those men doing," asks Susan.

"They are digging for clams and mussels buried in the mud."

"Oh," says Susan, who's probably pretty much a city girl from Philadelphia. At first, she's a little squeamish about getting her sneakers wet and muddy, but when she sees me actually skating across the slimy mud, she eagerly tries it, too.

"If you keep your feet moving, they won't get stuck. If you stand still, you can sink in pretty deep," I warn. She follows my advice.

Just ahead, Abigail cries, "Help, my shoe is stuck!," Mark, Sam, and Darryl try to help. They sink in the mud, too. The picture of the four trying to keep their feet moving, as they tug on the sunken shoe is priceless. They finally accomplish their task and move on to more solid ground.

Eddy splashes Kevin. Kevin splashes Eddy, and the water fight is on. The water's cold, as Maine ocean water always is. Several of the kids run into the water up to their knees. Jeff, Kyle, and Peter splash one another, laughing and squealing. I head away from the splashers. Susan follows.

"You sure like purple, don't you," I say.

"It's my favorite color, and all my relatives send me purple clothes and things. My grandmother gave me these pants."

"They're wild," I reply, and so are her purple shirt, headband, and purple rimmed glasses.

"And just how long have you loved purple, my dear?" I ask in a psychiatric voice.

"Oh, I don't know," she laughs. "You're funny, Dr. MacCracken."

Her parents, Brent and Marjorie, walk behind us. Brent takes a few snapshots of Susan and me. Soon they catch up.

"How are you doing, Susan," says her father. "This is certainly different, isn't it?"

"It's fun," she says. "Did you see me skate on the mud?"

We walk along together. Brent and I talk about the University of Pennsylvania where I went to medical school and where he has taught math for twenty years.

Pat and the others gather around the big rock. Tim waves to us to come over that way. I bet it's picture time. We always try to get a group photo on this rock. The kids climb up on top, and the parents surround the bottom. In my backpack I locate my little camera with a time delay, so I can get into the picture. We take turns posing and snapping. It's too bad Lydia and Nancy won't be in the group shot, but it's just the perfect weather and location for our picture.

We stop hiking and start playing. Mark and Peter begin a rock skipping contest. Eddy helps Tate look for more crayfish under the seaweed. Little Lucy and Emily fill their buckets with shells and pretty rocks, as Sam and Pearl look on. Becky and Ginny talk away from the group. Others chat while some just sit on the warm rocks and breath in the sea air. There's not a cloud in the sky.

My mind drifts back to other years here. Each year is different—and yet so much the same. I regret we haven't kept up with all the old campers, especially the ones from out of state. It's like they drifted into our lives, made a lasting impression, and then drifted back out. Occasionally, we receive Christmas cards from some. Most write to us the first summer after camp, but a few we haven't heard from since they drove out the driveway.

We've had some families come back after several years away. The children had grown and wanted to return. I'm not sure the second time is quite as special for them; it's like going back to your old college. Some of the old professors are still there, but without the friends that you met and cared so much about, it's just not the same. We tried to have alumni return for the Friday afternoon games and picnic. But that didn't work. It just put strangers in the midst of a newly formed close knit group. But, some day we'll have a reunion and communicate again with all these special folks.

"If you're ready for a snack, come on over," Pat calls. "It's about that time, and then we should be heading back."

The wind picks up, as it always does in the afternoon. We need to start back before the tide comes in too far. "All trash in this bag and we'll get going," I say. "Let's see if we can get back in time for the water slide."

"I'll beat everyone," says Jeff, as he heads toward home. Kyle is right behind him.

"No use going too fast. Pat and I will have to be there before you can start."

"Then, hurry Dr. Mac!" They still run ahead.

I notice Becky, Ginny, and Cindy walking together. Girl talk, I suppose. Perhaps Ginny can be positive role model for both of them. Tim and Darryl are talking, too. I pass them and overhear them discussing Becky's attitude and Nancy's depression. I catch up with Kevin, who is strolling back on his own. His jeans are soaking wet, but it doesn't seem to bother him.

"Kev, are you cold?" I say to start a conversation.

"Not really. What's the water slide like, anyway?"

"It's fun. You sit down on a plastic runway, we run water down the plastic, and you slide all the way to the bottom of the hill. It'll be good for you to have your jeans on. With only a bathing suit, sometimes kids burn their bottoms."

He smiles, "Thanks for the warning."

"Kevin, I want to talk to you about all these hospitalizations you've been having. Your mother's quite upset, and your case worker's concerned. And you've been missing a lot of school, too."

"I know. Mrs. Williams, my teacher, is afraid I'm not ready for seventh grade."

"Would that be a new school?"

"No, we go up 'til eighth in this school."

"Do you have any idea why you keep getting sick?"

"Mom, says it's 'cuz I'm sneaking food at school. Her friend saw me buying a Milky Way one day, so she thinks I do it all the time—but I don't. Well, not as often as she thinks."

"That might make you run high blood sugars, but it probably wouldn't be enough to get you into the hospital. Usually it takes infections, stress, or a lack of enough insulin to get you sick."

"Well, I got stress, that's for sure!" He splashes for a few steps.

"Is it school?" I ask, knowing that's not it.

"Not really. I have more trouble at home."

"With your sister?"

"Naw, she ain't bad really. It's my mom's new boyfriend," he says, with disdain. "He thinks he knows everything, and he don't know nothin'. I can't believe my mom wants to marry him. What a jerk!"

"Sounds like you have some pretty strong feelings about him. Does Cindy feel the same way?"

"I don't think she really likes him, but she says Mom is happier when he is around, so she thinks that's better."

"Is that true?"

"Well, she does make herself look better now. Before, she didn't care how she looked, but with me in the hospital so much, she hasn't been that happy."

"Can you blame her? Nobody wants their son sick in the hospital. She'd be a lot happier if you stopped getting sick."

"Yeah, and . . . "

"And what?"

"And she'd have more time to be with him, too." Kevin kicks the water again. He may have just realized that he has given himself away.

"Have you ever not taken your insulin when you were supposed to?" I don't wait long for his answer. "I've known a few kids who have occasionally skipped their shot to see what happens. Or sometimes to get into the hospital to get attention. It's a dangerous thing to play with your body like that. But it sure can be effective." I say no more. He's been listening.

"But, Dr. MacCracken, you'd think Lou was a jerk, too!"

"Well, I might, but that still doesn't make it safe or right for you to mess around with your insulin shots. There're other safer ways to communicate your feelings. In fact, I strongly recommend that we try to get you, your mom, and Cindy talking. Maybe Dr. Rogers could meet with you this summer."

"Dr. Rogers is okay, but that won't change my opinion of Lou."

"Just promise me you'll stop making yourself sick by skipping your shots. Believe me, that isn't going to solve anything, and you may get really sick or even be taken away from your mom." He looks up at me.

"That's not what I want."

"Well, you better keep yourself out of the hospital for awhile. I know you can do that, if you try." I put my hand on his shoulder.

"Yeah, I can."

"Good!" We both nod our heads in agreement. Maybe, he'll try it for awhile. I'm sure counseling can help, and if Tim thinks it helpful, maybe Lou could join the family sessions. Like Kevin, many kids have a hard time accepting their parent's boyfriend or girlfriend or later, stepparent. But the children with diabetes have dangerous and manipulative ways to show their objections.

Sometimes, the frequent hospitalizations occur because the child skips shots. But others can get so stressed by the emotional social situations that their bodies produce large amounts of stress hormones which counteract the metabolic effects of insulin. These are not easy kids to help and a great amount of time and energy goes into trying to stop the frequent hospitalizations.

Every diabetologist cares for a few kids who require multiple hospitalizations because of *ketoacidosis*—a metabolic state of insulin deficiency, either actual deficiency from not getting a dosage or two, or relative, with other hormones counteracting the insulin. Rarely, will the child admit to not taking his or her insulin.

I had one patient who returned as a young adult to see me. Several years before, I had spent at least two years trying to prevent his hospitalizations. When he returned to visit, he admitted to me that during those episodes, he had not been taking his insulin. He said he was trying to get back at his father who was an abusive alcoholic, and he found the hospital a friendly and safe place.

Another patient I cared for was sick almost every three weeks. In the hospital her blood sugars were still fairly high. She was withdrawn and uncommunicative. When asked about her diabetes, she'd say, "It doesn't bother me," and then be silent. She was a teenager who kept her feelings in. Educational testing showed us that she could only read on a third-grade level, yet was in regular eighth-grade classes. Can you imagine the stress of school. Once her school situation was rearranged, the hospitalizations stopped.

A few university centers have started long-term residential homes for these chronically sick children with diabetes. These children have emotional problems that play havoc with their diabetes. Luckily, the vast majority of kids with diabetes do very well. Some are never hospitalized after the initial diagnosis. From my experience and others, a stable family environment makes a big difference.

While Kevin and I talk, the tide creeps in. The others gather at the mouth of the little stream, which is now about two feet deep. It can reach waist height at high tide. For Little Lucy and Emily, it is very deep. Mark, Darryl, and Brent form a human chain, passing the little girls across the stream. Peter, Jeff, and Kyle are well ahead of the rest of the group. Those wearing bathing suits wade in deep and manage to get across with the steady hand of Eddy, who is on the other bank.

Sam lifts his mother in his arms and walks across the twelve foot stretch. To be chivalrous, Brent does the same for Marjorie. Becky, Ginny, and Cindy go further upstream and cross with little trouble. Kevin and I wade in, too. His jeans are already soaked, and my shorts barely get wet as I tiptoe across. A few others follow. Mark assists Big Lucy, who has been watching from the bank, obviously wondering if she can make it. With her limp, she might lose her balance in the slick sand.

Last to cross are Pat and Heather. They have been assisting everyone else, and the water level is rising. Mark, with his bathing suit on, and Tim, still quite dry, offer to piggyback these two lovelies across. They are delighted. Pat's backpack gets handed across first and then she gets on Mark's back. Heather whispers something into Tim's ear, as she climbs on his back. I tell Brent to get his camera ready, for I suspect a good photo opportunity here. My little camera is ready, too.

As Tim and Mark walk into the deepest part of the stream, Heather grabs Pat's shirt and says, "Let's see who can knock who over." At first, Mark looks surprised, but with the cheers from the dry bank, he takes the challenge. Tim has pulled this stunt before.

"Take them down, Pat!" I yell. Pat and Heather hold on to each other's arms, and the men circle round. Tim stumbles, tries to regain his footing, but the shifting of their weights causes the foursome to all fall down. And wet, laughing souls they are, too. As the four sea monsters stand, I snap their photo. A good one for the album.

I'm not sure the campers can quite believe that Pat, Tim, and Heather would do such a thing. But that's what makes this camp such fun. The staff's fun loving. And Mark's a prankster too.

Back at the lodge, Jeff is first in line for the water slide, which has been part of our camp from the beginning. Fearless kids love to squeal as they fly down on their rumps. We try to avoid the head first method, but several kids do helicopter turns on their bottoms, so you can't tell what's coming down first. The grass on the hill is mowed, and the plastic sheets are about four feet wide. Each year the run gets longer. I'd estimate this year it's about one hundred feet, ending in the tall grasses.

I vividly recall a few courageous moms taking their turns. I can't forget their surprised expressions. Sometimes, two or three campers slide together, as you would on a toboggan, but here there is no sled, just bottoms. The ground's a little hard and rough for my old spine. I stay at the bottom and monitor the children's safe landing, and that's just fine with me.

Pat runs the hose at the top. The plastic must be wet all the way down before the slide works well. At first the line of campers at the top is short. I guess Jeff will have to demonstrate first, before there's great enthusiasm. Tim, Darryl, and Lisa stand along the sides of the slide. Eddy, Sam, and I secure the bottom. Brent, located near the bottom, prepares his camera.

"Are you ready down there?" Pat yells.

"Ready!"

Pat wets down Jeff's bottom. You go faster with a wet rump. The hose gives a continuous stream. "Here I go," Jeff shouts. And he leans back shooting like a rocket down the plastic runway. He has learned the proper technique and flashes a big smile at the end of the run. Quickly, he charges up the hill for another turn.

The waiting line at the top increases. Kyle is next. Sitting up for his first run, he goes a bit more cautiously than his brother. But, still he smiles at the end. In turn, most of the kids try. Little Lucy looks like she wants to go, but hesitates for a moment. She grabs her father's hand, probably asking him to go with her. After Pat wets his bottom, Mark flops down, and Lucy jumps in his lap. On her way down Little Lucy's face expresses sheer joy—or is it utter fright. It isn't quite apparent whether she is going to cry or laugh at the bottom.

"Great job," says Eddy, who catches them. He must have noted the same fear in Little Lucy.

"Lucy, you were great!" I add. And she smiles a little.

As Mark gets up, he whispers in my ear. "Now I know why you stay at the bottom of the hill. Smart thinking, Doc." I smile. He's quick to discover my secret.

"Hurry up down there!"

"Out of the way!" the kids yell.

Up and down they go. We watch all different techniques of sliding, turning, and twisting. Around 4:30 when I start to see blue lips on some of the kids, I figure we better dry off and check blood sugars. "One last run!" I yell up to Pat. There's is a moan from the top of the hill, but the kids know I mean it.

Last one down is Little Lucy on her own. She has conquered her fear and I'm sure will be ready for the water slide the next time. For those campers who didn't try, like Sam and Emily, there will be another time.

"Susan's acting strange!" yells Tate, as he comes running out the door. "She's not talking right."

Susan's parents, Pat, and I run up to their room. Sitting on her bed, Susan just stares at the window. Her wet bathing suit is half way off. "Susan, it's your father, are you OK?" He shakes her.

"I'd like some mustard, please." She slurs the words.

"What's she talking about," says her mother. "Is she having a reaction?" Marjorie looks at me.

I pull out the tube of glucose gel I always carry in my pocket. "Here, Susan, here is your mustard," I squeeze the gel into her mouth. She slowly swallows it. "That's a girl, have some more." Her face is very pale, and the ring of white around her nose and mouth is unmistakable to Pat and me. This is low blood sugar, *hypoglycemia.* She had been very active on the water slide. Brent had taken several pictures of her sliding. Marjorie had commented to me that it was the most fun Susan has had in a long time.

"Susan, just relax. You're going to be fine. Your blood sugar is too low, and this will bring it up," I calmly suggest. Sometimes when people with diabetes have a reaction they refuse to eat or drink anything. They may insist nothing's wrong. If you try to force something into their mouths, they may clench their teeth. Luckily, Susan is quite cooperative in taking her "mustard." The low blood sugar in the brain causes confusion, and with that, the speech and thought pathways are disturbed. Who knows why she thought of mustard.

I should have been more on top of this. With all the extra exercise of the mud hike and then the water slide, I should have encouraged her to get a bigger snack. But we tell parents that hindsight must be used to educate, not to criticize or self-flagellate. I suppose I should take that advice, but my previous suspicion that she was on too much insulin should have been enough for me to watch closer.

Susan looks better. The blank stare is gone, as is the pallor. Tate, who has been nervously watching all of this, relaxes. It's very scary to watch someone have a reaction. Luckily, he noticed that something was wrong in the beginning. Susan remembers nothing of what she said, but admits she's hungry. Pat gives her half a granola bar, which she quickly inhales. We leave the family in their room and suggest that they get her into some dry clothes and then check her blood sugar. I ask Brent to talk to me before they give her any pre-supper insulin.

Pat and I go back to our cabin to change. My wet sneakers have about rotted my feet. Dry socks feel good.

"That was a strange reaction," says Pat.

"Yeah, sure glad Tate called us before she got any worse. I hate dealing with the big ones." She and I recall the only time we had a child have a seizure at camp. We hope to avoid that this year.

By 5:15 everyone's dressed. Word of Susan's episode has spread to the other parents and kids. Most of the blood sugars on the kids are within the normal range, lower than yesterday afternoon's readings.

"Jeff is always on the go," says his mother. "He rides his bike, plays soccer, and wrestles with his dad a lot. This was not a particularly unusual day for him. That's probably why he doesn't require much insulin."

"Anyone on the go like that will definitely require less insulin," I comment.

She adds, "I'll bet Susan is not very active at home. Her parents say she reads books all the time. Too bad she doesn't keep up with her little brother. Tate is quite a ball of fire. Jeff and Kyle think he is amazing."

I try not to discuss campers with other campers. But I love to hear their impressions. Many times it helps to substantiate my own. Having six families together for a week is very unusual. Various personality types emerge, as well as different ways of handling diabetes. As they share with each other, they'll see that there are different responses and answers to the same problems. Susan's hypoglycemic episode gives everyone a chance to think about what could have been done differently to avoid it, and what they would have done to treat it.

Pearl comes over to me to tell her story. Lydia and Nancy are standing nearby. "I'll never forget the time Sam was in bed and started screaming. Ollie, my husband and Sam's step-father, and I awoke from a deep sleep. Sam had only had diabetes about two months. We didn't know what was going on. He was thrashing all over. The ambulance is twenty miles away, but I called them anyway. Ollie held onto Sam, so he wouldn't hurt himself. We got just a little honey in his mouth. That's what our doctor had told us to use. After about ten minutes, well it seemed that long, he stopped and slowly opened his eyes. He didn't know where he was . . . thought he was back in the hospital. Gosh, were we scared. But when the ambulance arrived, Sam was fine. He was eating a big tuna sandwich. I can remember the look on that driver's face. Bet they must've driven a hundred miles an hour."

"But if he hadn't come out of it, you would have been mighty glad they'd come," Lydia comments.

"Yes," says Nancy, "You were right to call. I sure would have."

Pearl continues, "Sam admitted he had had some beers with his friends after a basketball game and had skipped his evening snack. We all learned later that alcohol can cause your blood sugar to drop, not rise. He didn't touch a beer again for a long time."

"After a tough basketball game, he probably could have used more calories, too," Nancy adds, looking over to me for approval. I nod.

I notice Brent standing a little bit away from me. He's holding an insulin syringe in one hand and two bottles of insulin in the other.

Recalling that I had wanted him to check with me before giving Susan her shot, I excuse myself.

"How is she?" I ask.

"Well, her blood sugar is now 230, so I thought I'd better give her some extra regular according our sliding scale."

I wince. I just hate that word "sliding scale." It's a term commonly used to describe a method of deciding insulin dosages by a fixed program according to the current blood sugar level. It's used a lot in hospitalized patients . . . orders left with the nurse, so the doctor would not have to be contacted for a decision, especially in the middle of the night. It might go something like this: Give 5 units for blood sugar below 150, give 6 units for 150 to 250, give 7 units for 250 to 350, etc. Of course, there are so many problems with this method that I hesitate to start to explain it to Brent now. Susan needs her insulin before supper, so I'll keep this brief. Tomorrow morning I'll speak to all the parents about a "sliding scale."

"Brent, the high sugar she has now is probably a combination of the glucose gel and granola bar we gave her, as well as her own body's response to the low blood sugar. It's a bit of a rebound, and I wouldn't be too concerned about it. What have her morning blood sugars been running since you've been here?" We turn around and look at the charts on the wall. Susan has kept very accurate records. "On Monday morning her blood sugar was 130 and this morning it was 235."

"I gave her more insulin this morning because of that high sugar, and our sliding scale suggests extra for anything over 200."

I say, "So today she's had more exercise than usual and more insulin, too. What are her usual morning blood sugars? Does she ever wake up with headaches?"

"Usually her morning sugars are fine—in the range of 70 to 100, but she does sometimes have unexplained high readings. Susan's always been prone to headaches, but her mother gets migraines, too. I'd guess a couple of times a week she has morning headaches. Sometimes she just doesn't want to get up. But I know she's not enjoying her teacher this year. Her teacher says Susan daydreams all the time."

Her symptoms of headaches in morning, not being too alert on rising, and the daydreaming in class could all be due to low blood sugars. She may be so tightly controlled that she's almost always on the border of a reaction or recovering from one. It reminds me of another little girl we had at camp. We were able to cut her total insulin dosage in half while she was here. She became a different kid, too. So much more energy and spirit. Sometimes, I'm afraid we create walking zombies with the overzealous approach to strict blood sugar control. There's no doubt, though, it's very tough to find the middle road.

"I would recommend cutting back on her insulin. I think she shows many signs of frequent undetected low blood sugar. Why don't you give her two units less of the regular tonight and two units less of the NPH. That's about a ten percent reduction and should be fine."

Brent heads back upstairs to find Susan.

Pat walks over to me. She's been checking some of the injection techniques of the kids and parents. She likes to watch how each child with diabetes gets or gives the injection. Often, she's able to pick up on some technical problems.

"You look heavy in thought," she says.

"Yeah, I guess so. I'm concerned about Susan."

The bell rings for supper. Jeff, Peter, Kyle, and Tate race down the driveway. The two little girls walk over, holding hands. Still carrying on their conversation on low blood sugars, Nancy, Pearl, and Lydia head for dinner. Abigail grabs Pat's and my hands and says, "Are you coming? Let's go eat." We three skip to supper.

■■■■■■■■■■■■■■■■■■■■■

C H A P T E R   7

A Long Day's Journey

The din in the dining hall is good to hear. Everyone seems to have something to say to someone. Today has been busy. The feelings session, the mud hike, the water slide, the reaction. All this breaks down the barriers; strangers are becoming friends. Just two suppers ago this room was quiet, and campers sat with their families, not knowing how to start conversations or what to talk about after the introduction. Tonight there's abundant conversation. I just wish I could hear them all.

Pat announces the evening program. First, the parents watch a movie, while the kids see and maybe create a puppet show. Then the kids will see a movie, while the parents talk some more. Eddy announces that right after supper he and Mark will organize an informal softball game for any who want to play. The evening is beautiful, and it's the longest day of the year.

Heather, Tim, Pat, and I stroll over to the cabin for a few minutes break. Tim can stay through the evening meeting. Heather says she'd like an opportunity to be with the parents. We decide that Tim and Heather will watch the movie with the parents, and then later we'll all join the parents, when the kids watch their movie. Becky, Cindy, and Kevin should watch the adult movie. We have a great movie for the younger kids.

Pat and I grab the puppets and start joking around. "Hi, I'm Doctor Lion, what's your name? "

"I'm Biff, and I have diabetes." Biff is a gray floppy donkey with the biggest eyes and ears. He knows a lot about diabetes, because he has had it now for years. But, when he first came down with it, he was really confused. Pat and I love to play with the puppets. There are even two puppet pancreases made of polka dot material. One has red buttons—those are beta cells that make insulin. The other pancreas has no red buttons, thus no beta cells and no insulin. The kids catch on to this quickly with the illustrated pancreas. A clever woman, Larrene Hagaman of Missouri, created this puppet set, and Pat and I have had lots of fun creating our own scenarios. The kids love to invent their own plays, too.

"Do you think the parents can handle the movie?" Heather asks.

"Well, they shared a lot of emotions this morning. Some were quiet, though, just listening. Maybe these folks will find it easier to talk about the movie. It usually stimulates discussion. And even if they don't like the movie, they can tell us why and that's often quite revealing," I say.

"Becky and Kevin will be able to relate to the angry teenager in the movie, and Sam might see himself in that actor who at first didn't want anyone to know he had diabetes," Pat says.

She and I have seen Pyramid Films' "Focus on Feelings" so many times, we know all the characters. We definitely get different responses to the movie from our campers, but we always get responses. And then we just go from there. One year we eliminated the evening session completely, because we felt everyone was exhausted from the morning's sharing. But, this year we agree to show the movie.

Grabbing our props, we head over to the lodge. An active softball game is going on. Eddy's team needs two more runs to tie the score. Peter's on second and Eddy's up. Two outs. Mark pitches the ball. Eddy swings and hits that ball half way to Boston. Peter, then Eddy, cross home plate, the rest of the team slapping their hands. A pop fly caught by Lydia makes the final out. Mark and Eddy call the game a tie, and the crowd heads to the lodge.

Emily and Little Lucy are swinging on the swingset half way down the field. Sam and Lisa push them. Sam seems more relaxed, though he isn't talking in the group much. I'm delighted he acknowledged that he had diabetes. That was obviously a real barrier that he had to surmount. After a few more pushes, the foursome climb up the hill.

As the group gathers in the hallway, we ask Kevin, Cindy, and Becky to sit in with the adults. They don't seem to mind. Perhaps, they like being treated like adults. The counselors will watch the movie, too. Tim leads the adults into the meeting room. It's great to have him here.

After setting up the nice wooden puppet stage, Pat calls the group together. Several ask about the movie, and Pat explains that it will be shown after our puppet show. They accept that. We first act out Biff's first day in the hospital. Biff, the donkey with long gray ears, has just come to the hospital. Dr. Lion tells Biff about diabetes. Using the two pancreases, with and without red buttons, the doctor teaches Biff what has happened to his own pancreas.

"I see," says Biff, after Dr. Lion's explanation. "All you need to do is sew my red buttons back on."

"I wish I could do that," says Dr. Lion, "but we will replace what the red buttons make with the insulin we give you."

Peter and Jeff remember their first day in the hospital. Little Lucy and Emily are more fascinated with the curtains and the puppets, than the plot. Abigail, Tate, and Peter decide they want to put on a skit. They're are born actors. They act out a reaction. With a little lamb puppet, Abigail plays the nurse. Peter is Dr. Lion. Tate is Biff, the hospitalized child with diabetes. Tate has seen his sister have many reactions and knows just what to do. The audience, which is Emily, Susan, Jeff, Kyle, and Little Lucy watch carefully, intrigued by the voices and action. The puppets jump all around the stage. After the patient is revived by the nurse and doctor with a pretend bucket of water with sugar in it, the young audience applauds wildly.

"Why don't you plan to give a little play for the talent show. We need good acts."

"Yeah, that would be fun," says Tate.

Emily and Little Lucy put the puppets on and dance them across the stage. Somehow these puppets almost come alive.

Tim rolls the TV and VCR out of the meeting room. It's time to set up the kids' movie. Becky and Kevin come out and ask if they can stay with the kids. Actually, that'll be fine because Kevin's mom and Becky's parents will be less inhibited with their children out of the room. As the movie begins, Emily climbs into Becky's lap, and Little Lucy sits with her brother, Peter. Pat and I join the parents in the other rooms.

"Anybody care to comment on the movie?" Tim asks.

Nancy starts, "I thought it was good. Becky could have played the angry teenager. I guess it's pretty common for kids to fight it."

"The teenager in the movie came around just a little bit in the end," says Marjorie. "I got the feeling there was hope there. Certainly, she wasn't quite as upset after hearing the other people talk."

"The moderator did an excellent job," states Brent, with an analytical tone.

And Brent is quite right. The moderator, Noreen Papathiodora, a well-trained, sensitive medical social worker, has had diabetes since she was a child. She empathizes with the group, and does a great job.

The telephone rings. Closest to the door, I run to answer it. The reporter from the *Bangor Daily News* wants to come down tomorrow afternoon to talk with the campers and take a few pictures. I explain that Wednesday afternoon is our free day, and most everyone will be out of camp. Could she possible come on Thursday. She thinks so, depending on the labor dispute at the mill. Then, she asks me directions, and what seems like a thousand other questions. I certainly want an article in the paper, but hate to be missing the discussion in the other room. For several years we haven't had any newspaper write-ups, but because this is our tenth year, she thinks it would be newsworthy. I close with, "Be sure to make that final right turn, at the second stop sign. See you Thursday."

As I walk by, the kids are laughing at the movie. No problems there. I return to the meeting room. Marjorie is wiping her eyes with a tissue. Everyone is engrossed. They hardly notice my return.

"It really helps to hear others voice some of your feelings and concerns," says Nancy. "That black woman said the same thing that I did this morning. She said she cried and cried. I guess I wasn't such an odd ball to be crying so much. Somehow, just knowing that makes it a little better."

Eddy speaks up. "The guy who was the actor and learned to tell his producer how to treat an insulin reaction seems to have accepted his diabetes pretty well."

"Yeah, but it took him awhile before he wanted to tell anyone," says Darryl.

Mark looks upset. "It was hard for me to listen to the guy who started to cry, saying he just didn't want to be different from others. That made me think about Peter. I try really hard to treat him the same as others. I want Peter to know that he can do anything he wants to, and others shouldn't treat him differently. But probably, I'm being a bit unrealistic. Even if I don't treat him differently, others will. And, maybe I need to face the fact that he is different. I mean his pancreas doesn't work, as it should. That's the only difference. So maybe I need to admit that he is different, but that doesn't imply that he is less able to do those things that he has a mind to. Maybe I, as the parent, just don't want to admit that my child has a defect." He stops.

Ginny is next to Mark. Her eyes reveal her concern. She speaks. "Peter is different in many ways from other kids. He's an unbelievable athlete for his age and much more developed than many ten year olds. Emily is different from every other kid here; she has red hair. I guess what I believe with the help of my uncle is that everyone is different from everyone else. It is funny, but having diabetes here at this camp makes you the same as many other kids.

I know it's hard to be different, but so do most kids in junior high who all yearn to be the same. But, just like the social scene gets easier as you leave junior high and enter high school, I mean, there's less emphasis on fitting in, so does diabetes get easier with time. A lot of times I forget I even have it."

Ginny's great, but not all see it her way. I hope her positive outlook continues. I'm sure at some point in her life she may get discouraged, but other adults with diabetes have told me that those moments of discouragement become fewer and fewer, and you do learn to go on with your life. For now, though, it's helpful to have her voice of optimism. If Sam would talk honestly, we might hear a harder story.

Lucy, who has been fairly quiet, comments, "I liked the moderator's remark about being in a boat on the stream of life. She said you could drift with the current or you could pick up the oars and row the boat. Researchers keep improving our oars and maybe they'll even find a motor to attach to our boat for improved performance." Her eyes twinkle.

"Yeah, I agree with you, Lucy," Lydia says, "that was a good comment. I hope Kevin can safely paddle his boat, someday." The other parents nod in agreement. The analog of actively working for health is helpful.

No one says anything for a few seconds. The movie served our purpose. The group has aired a few more feelings and restated a few from this morning. I'm pleased.

Tim closes. "I just want to say that I have enjoyed being with you all today. I'll be heading back to Bangor tonight. Wish I could stay and get to know you all better. If I can help any of you at any time, please give me a call. You can reach me through Pat or Dr. MacCracken at the Medical Center. I'm sure you'll have more opportunities to share this week. That's the important part. You all have a lot to teach each other, and you can all give each other wonderful support that is sometimes hard to find outside a community like this."

"Thanks for coming, Dr. Rogers," says Nancy.

"Thanks, Tim," adds Mark. The group gets up and stretches. Lydia goes over to Tim with a piece of paper and pencil in her hand. Maybe we can get them help. As the adults head out the door, the children's movie ends. Great timing.

A few of the kids are yawning. It's been a long day. Little Lucy is asleep on her brother's lap. He patiently waits for his father to collect her and take her upstairs. She hardly arouses. Victory over the water slide is exhausting. But, what a triumph!

The parents and Pat help the kids do their blood tests. I look over the results as the kids chart them on the bulletin board. Peter's is 90. I encourage him to eat a double snack. He's pleased with that. He isn't on much insulin in the evening, so he'll probably be just fine, but he was pretty active today, with several trips up and down the hill for the water slide after the mud hike and then some baseball after supper. Low blood sugar several hours after exercise can occur, so a double snack is a good idea, tonight.

Susan meticulously writes her value on her sheet and in her little book, too. She carefully uses the blue marker to indicate that the value is between 120 and 160. I just happen to notice that there are a lot of yellow values marked in her book. She tells me those are values under 80. But, tonight Susan's blood sugar is 117. That seems to be OK even with the two unit reduction in her regular insulin that I recommended to Brent. With two units less of NPH, the insulin that will work through the night, she should be fine. I'm sure she'll do so much better with less insulin.

I notice that Becky hasn't written down her blood glucose value for supper or bedtime. Nancy and Darryl appear to be backing off and not insisting on her recording the numbers. She's standing next to Ginny and Cindy near the piano. I interrupt their conversation, "Becky, have you done a test tonight?"

"Yeah, it was high again," she says with a discouraged voice, "and I didn't eat much supper either."

"If you record them on your chart, I may be able to help you make some decisions on changes you might need. Let's go write them in." She follows me, but I might as well be dragging her with a chain.

"Before supper I was 180 and now it's 298." She writes the numbers in pretty small, so they cannot be seen easily.

"Becky, last night your blood sugar was 165 at bedtime. Maybe tonight's high reflects the stress of the evening, especially if you say you ate a light supper. Did that movie bother you?"

"That movie got me mad, well, at least in the beginning. I feel just like that girl. I hate diabetes. And then it made me so sad watching that guy cry. Why do you show that movie anyway?" She looks right at me. Maybe she should not have watched it. But, I still think it helps these kids and parents to see they are not alone in their feelings of sadness and anger. "You should have a movie with just kids. There were too many adults in it for me."

"You're right. We need a movie just with kids. Pat and I plan on doing that sometime. Want to be a director or actress?" She looks at me with one of those slightly disgusted teenage glances. A classic. "Well, think about it. But, don't worry about your high sugar today. Emotions can really affect your level. Let's just see how tomorrow goes. If your sugars stay high, then maybe you should add more insulin."

Most everyone is heading upstairs. We say our goodnights and walk back to our cabin. Tim stays for a little while longer.

"What a day!" says Pat, as she falls into the stuffed green chair. She automatically picks up her knitting. Heather and I collapse on the old torn, but soft, couch. And Tim heads for the refrigerator.

"You guys have any Pepsi? I need caffeine for the drive back."

"We have diet Coke with caffeine. Will that do?"

"Sure, do you want anything?" He asks, opening his soda.

"No, thanks. I need a good night sleep. I'm mentally pooped." Tim gets comfortable in the wicker chair. "Tim, why don't you tell us your impressions," I request.

"Well, from my limited exposure of 12 hours or so, I'd say you have a few pretty depressed people here. And I know that's no surprise to you. Sam's depressed and from what you've told me he has reason to be. But I'm optimistic about him. This week will probably be the best thing for him. He may not participate much at first, but by the end of the week, I bet you'll see an improvement. His mother Pearl is a gem. Emily's irresistible, and she's really enjoying the other kids.

"That's for sure. She and Tate had fun designing their T-shirts this morning," Heather adds.

Tim continues. "I'm worried about Nancy. I didn't get to talk with her much, but Darryl spoke with me about her while we were on the mud hike. He blames himself for the problems at home and admits that he has run away from Becky's diabetes by becoming busier and busier on his sales route. And he knows Nancy is suffering, too. I guess she's seeing a counselor, but Darryl isn't sure that's helping much. He said sometimes he finds her at home just staring out the window. It seems she has lost most of her outside contacts because she tries to be home for Becky all the time."

Pat adds, "I talked with her some before supper. I wondered if her headache had gone away. She told me that when she gets upset, her headaches come on. From our brief conversation, I'd say Darryl and Nancy need joint counseling. Nancy implied she thinks Darryl has been seeing other women while he is off on his sales trips."

"Ah, the plot thickens," says Heather.

"I doubt that," says Tim. "I know I can be surprised just as others can about these things, but I would guess that's just Nancy's imagination and fear, as she sits home feeling more and more depressed. I think Darryl loves her but just doesn't know how to help either his wife or his daughter. And he'd rather hide from the problems."

"Well, that couple sounds desperate. How are we going to help?" Pat asks.

"It may be more than one week here can handle, though you guys have performed a few miracles I can recall," Tim quips.

"We do the best we can," I say. "What other jolly observations do you have for us, Dr. Rogers?"

"Well, Cindy and I had a long talk after lunch. She told me all about Kevin and his con games. She was pretty upset seeing her mom so distraught this morning. It really affects kids to see their moms cry. Cindy loves her mom, but they are really in a tight situation. They live in a space as large as my kitchen and family room. And you all know neither my family room nor my kitchen is large."

"Did she mention Lou, her mother's boyfriend?"

"Yeah. She isn't that unhappy about him. But he just might be their chance for a slightly better life," Tim adds.

"Kevin essentially admitted to me on the mud hike that he was manipulating his diabetes to get into the hospital," I comment. "I hope I successfully convinced him to stop playing those dangerous games. I'd better call his social worker. Could you see the family this summer if they can arrange transportation? If Medicaid won't cover their visits, maybe our special trust fund will."

"I think family therapy would help, provided they'll make the effort to come to Bangor."

Pat adds, "I think they will."

I glance at my watch. It's almost 10 o'clock. A 15 hour working day is long enough. Tim finishes his last swig of soda and rises to leave. "Well, thanks for the day. See you next week, and I'll be looking forward to hearing how things turn out."

"Thanks again for coming."

"Drive safely. There's probably some fog on the roads," I add.

"I will, and get a good night sleep," he says, as he closes the door behind him.

"Well, kiddos, what say we hit the hay? Tomorrow is another day." Heather is always full of these sayings.

"Pat, could you just clue me in on what goes on tomorrow?" She always keeps me on track. That's why she's the director and I'm the assistant director.

"Tomorrow, you take the parents in the morning and talk with them about hypoglycemia, at least that's the subject you told me you wanted to cover. You always do what comes naturally, anyway." She smiles. "You also wanted to cover *hyperglycemia*. I'll take the kids and teach them our skit on exercise. After snack, we'll present it to the parents. Heather has to go back to Bangor for a dietary

advisory meeting, and I'm sure she'll check in with her dog." Pat
smiles again. "You're leaving after breakfast, aren't you, Heather?"
Heather's in the bathroom, brushing her teeth. She grunts a muffled
"yes."

"Do you want to go to Fort Knox in the afternoon?" Pat asks
me.

"Sure, why not? I think I'll take Eddy and Ginny to Ellsworth
for a little break. But now I'm wondering if I should offer to take
Becky, too. That would give Nancy and Darryl some free time on
their own."

"MacCracken, you're a match-maker," Heather says as she
comes out of the bathroom.

"Well, they could probably use an afternoon together, alone.
And Becky might like to be with Ginny. Maybe some of Ginny's
positive approach could rub off."

"Sounds good to me," says Pat. "You can ask her in the
morning. We better get to bed." In less than a few minutes, I doze
off.

I awake abruptly to a crashing sound and then a male voice
calling, "Pat, Dr. MacCracken, come quick, Susan's having a bad
seizure!" Pat gets her light on before I do, and that light is enough
for me to find my jeans and sweatshirt. I quickly step into my boat
shoes, grab the glucagon kit, and charge out the door toward the
lodge. Pat and Eddy are right behind me.

The main lodge is still fairly quiet. There are lights on in the
Booth's bedroom. As I enter the room, I notice Susan on the floor
with her mother and father on either side. Tate watches from the
upper bunk. His sister is lying still now, but not arousable. Brent
tells me that she was shaking all over for several moments. Initially,
she let out a strange scream, and when they got the lights on, Susan
was on the floor. Marjorie says the shaking must have lasted ten
minutes, but Brent recounts it was probably closer to five. Either
way, to them, it seemed like an eternity.

Since she stopped thrashing, Brent has been squeezing small
dabs of glucose gel into her mouth. Some of the red gel is dripping

down her cheek. As they tell me the story, I draw up the *glucagon*, a hormone which will help Susan's body bring her blood sugar up. I only inject half the standard dosage to try to avoid the miserable side effect of vomiting. I can always give more, but usually the lower dosage works. Brent has probably gotten some sugar into her system. It's risky to give anything by mouth when someone is unconscious. You want to be careful that they swallow and not inhale into their lungs.

While we wait for the glucagon to work, I see fright on the faces of Susan's parents and brother. Luckily, I can't see my face. I try to remain cool and composed, but I too just hate this. It's frightening. I guess this is the worst reaction she's had. Brent says he's heard her cry out in the night before, but she's never had a seizure.

Pat suggests we get a blood test and has the machine ready to go. The blood glucose level should be rising now with the sugar Brent gave her by mouth, the glucagon injection in the arm, and her own body's response.

As the seconds count down for the machine's digital readout of the glucose level, we all watch Susan. She's so pale and clammy. But, she responds to her mother's soft voice and touch. The poor kid. No one should have to go through this. The poor family. And little Tate. He's only six. How frightening to see your sister like this. And it's all brought on by the medicine that is supposed to be the very treatment for diabetes. It's like walking a knife edge, trying to balance the blood glucose level. But we can't lose perspective of the whole child and family. If tightly controlled blood glucose levels are our only goal, then we'll run the risk of low blood sugars, and most probably seizures. For children, at least, I think that is too big a risk.

"Fifty-two," Pat says. It must be on it's way back up. Susan was probably in the twenties or thirties or maybe lower. The glucagon works quite rapidly, enabling the liver's storage supply of glucose to be dumped into the bloodstream. Its effect does not last very long. Either the injection must be repeated, or some food must be eaten.

Susan's eyes open now. She looks very confused. She'll have very little memory of the whole thing, but her family will never forget. Still saying nothing, she looks at her mother. Her father grabs her hand and gives it a squeeze. "How do you feel, honey?" he asks.

She replies slowly, "I'm hungry," and smiles faintly. What must it feel like to have five adults and your little brother all staring at you, as you lie on the floor. And she must be wondering how she got there anyway. Brent picks up his daughter and places her on their double bed. Marjorie pulls the sheet up.

"What would you like to eat?" her mother asks.

She opens her eyes again. Obviously, she is tired. "I'd like some Cheerios, please."

"Coming right up," Eddy says. He takes off down the stairs to go to the French House. Meanwhile, Pat has brought up a glass of apple juice from the refrigerator.

"Drink a little of this for me until Eddy gets back with your Cheerios." Marjorie helps hold the glass, but Susan readily drinks the juice. At least, so far, the glucagon has not made her nauseated. I think she's going to be okay.

Mark and Lisa, who have the room next door, come out to check on the commotion. Their three kids are heavy sleepers and have not been disturbed. Pat explains that Susan had a bad reaction, but everything is okay now. They go back to bed.

Eddy returns pretty quickly. A few Cheerios spill on the staircase, but most remain in the bowl. Susan's sitting up, ready for her snack. Tate, satisfied that she'll be fine, rolls over to go back to sleep. That's what a six year old should be doing at 1:30 in the morning. That's even what a 45 year old should be doing.

Pat rechecks the blood sugar. It's 110, and with the cereal it'll go even higher. But at this point we aren't as concerned about the high side. We just don't want it to drop again. I suggest that they check it again around 3:30 and feed her again, if necessary. I don't think that will be a problem. As we walk down the stairs, I comment to Pat, "I don't understand this. She got two units less regular and two units less NPH before supper. Can you imagine how bad the seizure would have been if she had been given four additional units?"

"The exercise today must have really been an unusual amount for her," Pat suggests.

Eddy heads back to bed, too. We thank him for being such a good messenger. He flew to our cabin and to the French House. And he has been emotionally stressed by this, too. We suggest maybe he should check his own blood sugar and eat something if he's low. He laughs, and says he feels fine, just understandably tired. He shuts his door. As we head for the outside door, Brent comes down the stairs. Both Pat and I turn simultaneously. Is Susan okay?

"Dr. MacCracken, Pat, could I talk to you for just a minute?" He looks drawn, exhausted. His blue bathrobe is disheveled, and his hair is standing straight up. He runs his hands nervously through his hair.

"Sure, let's go into the meeting room. Our voices won't carry in there." We walk through the swinging doors, and I find the light switch.

"There's something I have to tell you. I can't believe I didn't listen to you this evening. But I was so sure that she would need more insulin to cover that high sugar. I did give her one unit less of the regular, but I didn't change the dosage of NPH at all. I just thought she was doing OK with her morning blood sugars and didn't want her to get too high. Boy, was I wrong!" He buries his head in his hands.

"I just can't seem to make it work. It's so frustrating. There seems to be no rhyme or reason to her values. I've tried to learn everything I can about this. And complications really scare me. I want her blood sugars to be normal all the time. My wife always looks to me to make the decisions. She says I'm the mathematician. I've tried to talk to our doctor. Maybe some of his suggestions just aren't the best for kids. I don't think he sees too many children. I hope you aren't too mad at me. You certainly have a right to be. I'm really sorry—and sorry for Susan, too." Brent is very upset. Parents always live with the fear that their child might have died from the seizure, even though that's very rare.

"Brent, you did what you thought was best. She probably is on too much insulin and may have had the seizure even without those three extra units. She leads a fairly inactive life, reading her books. The exercise today with the mud hike, the water slide, and the baseball game may have been just too much for the insulin she's been on. She's going to be OK now. We can drop back on her insulin in the morning, and for the next few days try to determine a good dose for her. And in the morning we can talk more about realistic glucose levels in kids."

"Susan had so much fun today. She's really been happy here, and I think this exercise is good for her. I guess I just haven't had to put exercise into the equation of her control. Obviously, here I will."

"And that's what we are here for, to help you learn the fine tuning," Pat says.

And I add, "Brent, you're a good dad. Diabetes, unfortunately for all of us, doesn't fit too well into a standard equation. I sure wish it did. We just have to learn as many of the variables as we can, and I'm sure that still won't make it entirely predictable. But, it certainly will increase our chances for better control. Somehow we all need to remember that they must be treated as kids with diabetes, not diabetics who happen to be kids."

"That will take some adjusting on my part. I suppose I've been too caught up in the numbers." He looks up at both of us. Pat puts her arm on his shoulder.

"Try to get some sleep. Susan will be just fine. We'll see you in the morning." Brent heads up the stairs. The lodge is quiet.

He turns around and whispers, "Thanks, you two."

We whisper back, "Good night." I quietly close the front door. We walk back to our cabin in silence. It's times like these when you feel so helpless. There is a hurting man, a frustrated mathematician, a guilty father. Few people outside the grips of diabetes understand all this. What can we offer these families? Some education to help the frustration. I'm not sure that will do it. As Darryl said this morning, he would give anything for it to go away.

All the health professionals working in diabetes are hoping for a new, sophisticated prevention and cure. But, in the meantime, what can we offer? I guess we offer support—and sharing and understanding. Those of us not in research, not on the cutting edge of finding that cure and prevention, can help these families by giving them aid, comfort, and information until research makes our jobs obsolete.

"Pat, thanks for being here." I say. "We make a good team."

"Yep, and I couldn't do it without you," she responds.

"This may have been the longest day, but it feels to me like the longest night, too."

"You can say that again!"

And jokingly I do. "This may have. . . ." She gently shoves me in the back, as I open the door to the cabin. All is quiet in here, too.

"I'm beat," Pat sighs. Dropping her shoes on the floor, she crawls into her sleeping bag on the bed.

"Good night, see you in the morning." My room is cold, and so are the sheets. I find my wool socks and climb back into bed. I'm wide awake. Emergencies like that aren't too conducive to immediate sleep. I can't help but think about Brent, Marjorie, Susan, and Tate. And what about Sam and Kevin. Are we going to be able to have an impact on their lives? Can we help them handle their situations better? God, I hope so.

My mind drifts. I guess I do get involved with my patients. I reflect back to two incidents in my medical training. The first was when I was a fourth year medical student at the University of Pennsylvania. I went in to my advisor to find out my grade in my pediatric neurology elective I had completed. My advisor read to me the comments made by the chief of pediatric neurology. "Joan is an excellent student. She is competent and thorough. Her interest in pediatrics is apparent. She deserves an A. However, I must comment that I feel she sometimes gets too involved with the patients and their parents."

"Too involved," I thought. What does that mean? Does that mean that I shouldn't have spent so much time talking to that mother whose seven month old daughter was regressing in her development. The little girl could no longer sit up, and previously she had been crawling. This disease, Wernig-Hoffman's disease, is devastating, progressive, fatal. Perhaps because I hadn't seen many cases before, it hit me harder. Perhaps I hadn't developed the protective shield that most doctors supposedly need to survive. Is that what he meant? I really didn't know whether that neurologist was right or not. I suppose I should have talked with him, but I didn't. I remember my advisor, one of the few female internists on the staff, looked at me and said, "Joan, that's only one doctor's opinion. Follow your own instincts."

And so I have. As an intern, I took care of a young boy, ten or so, with leukemia. I'll never forget Vance. He was a terrific kid. One night he needed an x-ray, so I carried him on my back down to radiology. He held the requisition slip. It was a fun ride. Vance had many relapses of his leukemia. I kept track of him, even though I had changed services.

One day I heard he was being discharged and went to his room to say good-bye. As I entered the room, he moaned and said he had a stomachache. I pulled back the sheet to exam his abdomen and out popped one of those spring-coiled snakes. Scared me to death. Vance laughed and laughed. He died six months later. I had the opportunity to say a prayer at the bedside. His parents and I shared Christmas cards for many years after. And when they heard my first child was due on Valentine's Day, they wrote to say how delighted they were. That was Vance's birthday.

I do get involved, and it sometimes hurts to care. But, for me, it's the only way.

Rebounding and Dealing with Lows

Slowly I realize it's morning. The rain in my last dream is actually the sound of Pat's shower. My night's sleep, what there was of it, was filled with dreams of some of my old patient's from Denver and Boston.

"Your turn," Pat calls, as she comes out of the bathroom.

The shower revives me. Pat and I walk over together. Somebody has already started the coffee. Not too many of the campers are downstairs yet. As the week goes by, folks feel more relaxed and they take a few extra winks. I'm sure many are exhausted from yesterday. Tate could probably sleep all morning.

Wednesday, break day. After the first two years of running camp, we decided that everyone could use a break from the intensity of thinking about diabetes all the time. So we arrange the day to give families time to be together away from here, if they wish. For the past two years I've taken the counselors to Ellsworth to look around. Last night both Eddy and Ginny told me they'd love to go. Now, with my new plan, I'll ask them if it's okay for Becky to come.

Brent, with his cup of hot coffee, walks over to me and says

Susan was OK through the rest of the night. He checked her at 3:30 and she was fine. This morning her sugar is a little high, but he thinks it's because of all the food she had after her reaction. We carefully look over her chart again. She's had some type of reaction every day. Her lunch readings have been low. He says this afternoon they plan on driving to Blue Hill, about 15 miles away. They might climb the local mountain for the great view. Brent remembers strolling up that hill years ago with Marjorie. It's a moderate hike to the top.

"Susan will be pretty busy this afternoon, then." I say. "It sounds like a fun trip, returning to old stomping grounds. I think you could safely decrease both her regular and her NPH by 2 units. By my calculations, she's on more than 1 unit per kilogram and that's a hefty dose for a 10 year old. We might try to bring her down to about three quarters of a unit per kilogram and see if she stops having so many reactions. It's quite possible she'll feel more energetic, and she may be able to concentrate in school better next fall."

"OK, we'll try that." He looks at me, recalling our late night conversation. I ask him to be sure to tell Susan why we are doing this. She's still upstairs; otherwise, I would have her in on the decision making. Kids need to understand what goes into making a change in insulin dosage, for soon they should be making their own changes. But at this point I just need to gain Brent's confidence.

Emily, with her red hair in tidy little braids, is at the blood testing table next to Pat. On her tiptoes she watches as Jeff carefully pricks his finger. Emily is fascinated by Jeff, who is only two years older but must seem so much more grown up to her. Pat works with Jeff to be sure he has his technique down right. Then she'll teach him how to draw up his own insulin. That would make Jeff and his mother Lucy happy.

"Good job, Jeff," says Pat. "Excellent technique. You even remembered to wash your hands." Jeff grins.

"One hundred and one!" he shouts, obviously pleased. It's amazing how significant a number can be. With these machines with digital readouts, the kids lock onto the number. It's much more meaningful to them than trying to estimate a color chart, getting a range of blood glucose values, like 80 to 120. The first versions of these home blood glucose monitors were not very precise. The newer models have eliminated some of the possible user errors, like inaccurate timing and incomplete blotting with cotton. But they still have built-in error ranges of ten to fifteen percent.

Most kids believe the number to be exact. And they feel so badly when the value is high. It's like it's all their fault. Parents might say, "What did you eat? Are you telling me the truth?" We all wonder why a sugar is elevated, but there are so many variables. True, a candy bar inhaled in a moment of defiance will produce that hated high number, but so can an emotional upset or an insufficient amount of insulin. We try hard not to use the terms "good" and "bad." If you say that's a good value, then the opposite is a bad value. Most kids will unconsciously convert that into, " Then I'm a bad kid when I have a bad number." We try to say that's high, low, or in the normal range. But, it's easy to fall into saying "good" and "bad" because so many people use those terms.

Juggling his small soccer ball, Peter comes downstairs to check his blood sugar. He puts his ball down and tells Pat he just took a shower, so his hands are clean. She asks him to wash off at least one finger, because he has been playing with the ball. He does that in the nearby bathroom and then quickly pricks his finger. Emily is still watching. Peter puts the drop of blood onto the blood testing strip. With this machine there is no blotting at all. He talks to Jeff, who apparently wants to compare his value with Peter's.

The blood testing machines have been constantly changing since the first ones came out more than 10 years ago. I say more than 10 years ago, because we have never used urines at camp for checking these children with diabetes, except for looking for ketones. But sometime between the end of my endocrine fellowship at Boston Children's Hospital and the first few years of my practice here in Bangor, these machines started to be used by the people with diabetes.

The machines have gotten smaller and smaller. Some new models are shaped like pens, others are hardly bigger than a thick credit card. The finger prick contraptions are more gentle now and adjustable for various thicknesses of skin. And the methods of manipulating the blood glucose strips have changed, too. The old strips had to be rinsed after two minutes with water. One year a drug company donated these rinse bottles that had long thin plastic spouts with a pointed end. Two teenage boys here that year took great advantage of those bottles, making them into awesome squirt guns. And most of us got squirted at unexpected moments. They had a ball! It makes me smile just thinking about it. Anyway, strips don't need to be rinsed anymore, or blotted. Just a small drop of blood needs to be put on the strip.

"One hundred and eleven." Peter reads his value out loud. He is pleased with that. Both he and Jeff write their numbers on their charts.

Someone behind me says, "Dr. MacCracken." I turn. Sam must have been standing behind me for awhile. I was so interested in watching the kids with Pat that I hadn't noticed him. I suspect he was watching them, too. Both Jeff and Peter make it all look so painless and so matter-of-fact—just another routine, like brushing your teeth.

Sam continues, "I've been running pretty high in the mornings. Do you think if I start that night shot it will help?"

"I'm sure it will. Your morning NPH insulin doesn't last through the night. Most adults and older kids are on two shots, some three and some four times a day. A few very young children can take insulin only once a day, but generally that's an older mode of treatment that most physicians have dropped."

"Do you think I should use regular insulin, too."

"Yes. Just like Emily, you could use some short-acting insulin. I'm sure you'll have better control."

"Well, Mom says she wants me to learn about mixing the insulins because she's afraid if something happened to her, I would have to give Emily her shot. You know I just really didn't want to learn anything more. I was so mad about Emily getting diabetes."

"Well, Emily is taking quite an interest in all this stuff, so you're going to have to learn just to keep up with her." I smile and look over at Emily. She's still standing right next to Pat and watching Kevin do his test. It's always amazing to see how much these young ones learn by watching.

Sam and I decide on a dosage for him to start with. The beginning dosage is usually an educated guesstimate. We'll have to check his blood sugars frequently for the next few days to see if the dosages are close to being correct. Adjustments can be made up or down. I ask him to talk to Pat about the proper technique in drawing up two types of insulins. Sam goes over and waits in line with the other kids. Emily smiles, as she sees her father standing behind her.

More campers congregate downstairs. Several parents have their early morning coffee. Lydia, holding her coffee mug, has a white towel wrapped around her head. I overhear her talking to Big Lucy. Lou, her boyfriend, is coming up this afternoon to take them out. She thinks maybe they'll go up to the Bangor Mall. Her kids will probably like that. She says she hopes Kevin will be nice to Lou. They always fight. Lucy says her husband, Steve, is coming down for supper and the campfire. Her boys have been looking forward to seeing their dad.

"Ring the bell for breakfast," says Pat.

Jeff and Kyle both jump up on the bench. Jeff gives the rope a good tug, and Kyle gives it two more. Everyone gathers around as Pat makes her morning announcements.

"After breakfast the adults will meet with Dr. MacCracken to discuss low sugars, and the kids will meet with me to learn a skit about exercise. Why don't the parents meet in the group room, and we'll meet outside by the picnic table. This afternoon is free time to be with your family. We have several pamphlets on interesting sites in the area. If the weather stays nice, you may want to sunbathe on the beach. Just down the road is the town beach with a nice swimming area. Around 3 o'clock Dr. MacCracken and I will be going to Fort Knox, just down the road. If you want to come with us, you're invited. It's a fascinating place to explore. Bring a flashlight if you're coming. The tunnels are dark. And tonight we'll have a campfire down on the beach, weather permitting."

"What time will the campfire be?"

"We'll start around 7:30. Maybe a baseball game before."

"Yes!" says Peter. He's always up for a good game, soccer, or baseball or whatever.

"We're going to Blue Hill. Daddy, can we be back for the game?" asks Tate, who seems to have survived last night.

"We'll see," says his father.

"Let me add that it's time for you all to start thinking about the talent show for Friday night. Heather, Pat, and I are secretly practicing for our debut. Don't hesitate to sign up on the board. Any raw talent is accepted."

"Kyle and I know what we're going to do. We are . . . ."

Pat interrupts, "Don't tell us; keep it a surprise. Just let us know the name of your act."

"If there are no other questions, we better get to breakfast," Pat directs.

After breakfast, we grown-ups decide to walk down to the birch grove near the edge of the cliffs. Some sit on the rough wooden benches, while the rest of us sit on the grass. The sun's warm. It's a peaceful, quiet spot. I enjoy teaching here.

"I thought this morning we could talk about hypoglycemia—low blood sugar. First, I'd like to hear from you all what symptoms your own child shows when his or her blood sugar is low. Mark, what do you notice in Peter?"

"Um, Peter gets quiet, I'd say. He's so active that when he stops, I tend to think he's low, and he'll usually say he's hungry."

Lisa nods her head in agreement. She adds, "Sometimes, he gets a headache, but it goes away with milk or juice. He hasn't had too many lows."

"Peter has had diabetes only six months and is on a fairly low dose of insulin. He appears to still be in his honeymoon phase," I comment.

"Joan, could you tell me what that phase is again?" asks Lydia. "I don't remember if Kevin ever had that."

"It's a rather silly phrase, I guess. But the term 'honeymoon phase' describes that time after the diagnosis when very little exogenous (from outside the body) insulin is required, and the person's own pancreas is still able to make some insulin. It's something like a remission. During this time the blood sugars are fairly easy to control because of the endogenous (that means from within) insulin being made. The honeymoon period ends when the person's own pancreas is what we call, 'exhausted,' or doesn't make any more insulin. Then the insulin level is totally determined by the insulin that is injected (exogenous). And that makes control of blood sugar more difficult."

"I remember when Jeff was in his honeymoon phase. We almost had to stop his insulin completely. It was like his pancreas was almost able to make all the insulin he needed. I remember praying that his diabetes was going away, but you made me keep giving him just very small amounts and watching his sugars. It only lasted about three months, but then his insulin needs increased again," Lucy relates.

"It can be a hard time because on the one hand the diabetes is easy to control and yet the emotions of dreaming of possible permanent remission are hard to control. We teach parents that the honeymoon period can end slowly with a gradually, increasing need for insulin, or rather abruptly with a fairly sudden need for significantly more insulin. Probably everyone but Peter is out of their honeymoon."

"Does everyone have a honeymoon?"

"No, not everyone. But about 75 per cent of kids do. I think it depends on how long the diabetes has gone on without being diagnosed. If the diagnosis is made early, when there is a high sugar noted in a routine urine specimen or a little bit of excess thirst makes an alert doctor wonder about diabetes, these kids have not completely stressed their pancreas. Their honeymoon period may last quite a long time. But if symptoms have gone on for a long time and the child is really ill before the diagnosis, this child may have a shorter or even no honeymoon phase."

"That's what happened to Kevin. He was really sick."

"His honeymoon phase may have been short or nonexistent. Nancy, can you tell when Becky is low?"

"I used to think it made her irritable, but recently she's cranky a lot, and it can't always be low blood sugar. I guess sometimes she gets shaky and sweaty. She's pretty good, I think, at knowing if she needs something. But if I ask her to test to be sure, she just says, 'Mother, I know I'm low.' So, I have kind of backed off."

"Some kids do have pretty good internal radar to sense what their blood sugars are. At least they think so. But, repeated studies have documented that it actually is hard to tell where your glucose level is. That's why these little monitor machines can be a help— that is if the kids consider them as a help and not a pain in the neck."

"When Jeff was younger, he used to say 'I'm low' often. He knew he would get something sweet like a cookie. After awhile Steve and I caught on and started checking his sugar. Most of the time it was not low. So when it was low, we gave him milk instead of a cookie, and soon he stopped saying he was low all the time."

"Milk doesn't work for Kevin," Lydia comments. It's great to see her interest.

"Sometimes, if the blood sugar is really low, milk works too slowly. But, in general, it's a good treatment for mild reactions. We usually recommend 3 to 4 glucose tablets, if available, to prevent overtreatment," I add. I notice Marjorie taking notes.

"Pearl, can you tell if Emily is getting low?" Pearl has been rather quiet, but attentive. With Pearl and Sam sitting next to each other, I notice, for the first time, the resemblance. It would probably be more striking without Sam's red beard.

"Emily climbs into my lap, or onto our couch to lie down. I don't think she knows when she's low. She gets pale, too. Don't you think, Sam?"

Sam nods his head but says nothing else.

I continue. "It can be tough to tell when little children are low. Often they can be crabby, sleepy, or cuddly just because that's the way they feel at that moment. But other times these can be symptoms of low blood sugar." Several parents nod in agreement. I continue, "Sometimes, if the blood sugar is dropping rapidly, it can feel like your blood sugar is low. Also people with diabetes feel low blood sugar symptoms at a higher level of blood sugar than those of us without diabetes."

"That's interesting," says Brent. "You mean the level that Susan feels hungry and sweaty could be higher than when Tate or I would feel those symptoms?"

"That's right. We need to be aware of the values around 60 or 70. These levels can cause symptoms in your children."

"But sometimes Becky may be low, say 50 or so, and say she feels just fine. She's not always consistent in how she feels at a certain level," Darryl adds.

"That's true, too, and may have something to do with how rapidly they get to that level or whether they slowly drop over a fairly long period of time. Researchers are investigating these observations. You all recognize certain signs—paleness, lethargy, shakiness, headache, sweating, hunger, fussiness. Anything else?"

"Sometimes Susan just stares. Yesterday she said something that didn't make sense," Marjorie comments. "What was that she said? Oh yes, 'can I have some mustard?'"

I explain. "There are two groups of symptoms that can occur with low blood sugar. The first set of symptoms is brought on by the hormones, specifically epinephrine and glucagon, that are released in response to the low sugar. We call these 'counterregulatory hormones.' They counter or oppose the effects of insulin and cause the body to bring the blood sugar up.

"Symptoms that indicate these hormones are being released include those that occur in a fright or flight situation. You know, the way you feel when you look in the rearview mirror and see a police car with his lights flashing or when you see a moose charging at you. Your knees shake, you start to sweat, your heart races, and you are anxious and nervous."

Sam smiles. Perhaps he has been charged by a moose. "The other set of symptoms are due to *neuroglucopenia,* which is Greek for low glucose in the brain or nervous system. Without enough glucose going to the brain we can have sleepiness, headache, double vision, stubbornness, confusion, strange behavior, and poor coordination. Low blood sugar can impair abstract thought, like memory, calculations, or judgment. Still more severe would be seizure and coma. Usually, the first group of symptoms warns us that we need sugar. But occasionally the second set of symptoms occurs without early warning. It's important for everyone who is dealing with your children to understand all these symptoms."

"So it's possible that Susan's poor attention in class might be due to low blood sugar?" asks Marjorie. Brent nods. And I concur. Marjorie continues, "Her worst class is math, which is right before lunch. She probably is concentrating more on her hunger than her math."

Sam contributes, "I hate the feeling of low sugar. It's the worst. When I need to get something to eat 'cuz my sugar's low, I can't think about anything else, that's for sure. I usually feel like eating the whole refrigerator—and sometimes I do."

Pearls smiles. "That's true. He gets really hungry in the afternoon and eats half of my supper a few hours early."

I add, "Being on only one large dose of intermediate insulin in the morning, which peaks in the afternoon, could set you up for a reaction before supper. We'll be able to curb your Big Mac Attack by lowering your intermediate dose and adding regular in the morning."

"You're only on one shot a day?" asks Brent.

"Yeah, but I'm starting on two shots today," Sam says. He looks at me.

"We'll talk more about insulin and its action tomorrow. Let's get back to low blood sugars. I mentioned the *counterregulatory hormones,* like glucagon and epinephrine, that our bodies make in response to low blood sugar. I want to be sure you understand what I mean by 'rebound,' sometimes called the *Somogyi phenomenon.*

"When someone has a low blood sugar and these counterregulatory hormones are released, the blood sugar will rise. In those of us who do not have diabetes, insulin will be secreted if the blood sugar goes too high in response to these other hormones. But in a person with diabetes they depend only on the insulin that has been injected earlier. There will be no infusion of new insulin, and the blood sugar can go quite high.

"This is called a 'rebound.' It's a high blood sugar following low blood sugar. Actually, it's a survival mechanism to pull the sugar back up, but sometimes it will be too effective and you get high blood sugar (hyperglycemia). Does everyone understand that explanation?"

They nod. "I must tell you that some researchers feel we clinicians have made too much out of this rebound phenomenon. Some feel the rebound is usually due to overzealous treatment of the reaction. From my experience if you eliminate the lows, many of those highs that follow will go away. The fact that everyone feels low blood sugars slightly differently, and everyone reacts at slightly different levels, makes it very hard to predict.

"You parents will be the best primary physician for your own child. You're with them much more than your doctor, and you'll know the signs to look for in your own child. What you parents observe about your child's reactions is very important. With time, you should be able to notice subtle signs well before a casual observer, and you can then tell the teachers the specific signs and symptoms that your child experiences. Then they'll know what to look for.

"We have some excellent literature for the school personnel. The University of Michigan has put together a pamphlet we think all schools should have. It is entitled *Children with Diabetes: A Guide for School Personnel.* Maybe, you can encourage your librarian to get a copy for the school."

"Our assistant principal has a child with diabetes, and he has made sure the school system has books on diabetes," says Lucy.

"Do you have copies here?" asks Brent. I nod. Perhaps, he'll donate a copy to Susan's school.

"Let me summarize for a moment. Hypoglycemia occurs with two basic classes of symptoms, one from the production of counterregulatory hormones released in response to low sugar and, two, the direct effect of low blood sugar in the brain.

" The low blood sugar can be followed by a high blood sugar, even if it is not treated with food, because of the metabolic effects of those counterregulatory hormones. Different people feel low at different levels, and an individual, depending on many factors, may feel low at varying levels.

"Many people cannot sense low blood sugars very well. Low blood sugar should be treated as soon as it is recognized, preferably after a blood test to document it, but that is not essential. And food should *not* be withheld if symptoms point strongly to a reaction. Milk works well if the level is not too low.

"Other treatments would include quick sources of sugar. We think that the glucose tablets are handy to have for immediate consumption. If symptoms do not subside after 10 minutes, then the treatment can be repeated. It's good to proceed with a more substantial snack including some protein and fat, if a meal is not scheduled for awhile. I'm sure I've forgotten several other things I wanted to say. Does anyone have any questions?"

Brent clears his throat and asks, "Is there long-term harm in having hypoglycemic seizures?" His brow is creased with worry, as he nervously sits on his hands.

"That's a good question, and unfortunately I can't answer it completely. We don't know the long-term neurological effects of either severe, documented reactions or the silent ones that may go undetected.

"From surveys, we know that about 30 per cent of children with insulin-dependent diabetes mellitus have had severe hypoglycemia (seizure, coma, or both). And 22 percent have had more than one episode. So it's not a rare occurrence by any means.

"There are some studies done with younger children who had a history of frequent hypoglycemic seizures. Some of the children under age five at the time of the seizures were shown to have some learning difficulties later on. The growing brain, say before the age of two or so, is most susceptible to effects from frequent hypoglycemia. Pediatricians and pediatric endocrinologists have always been more concerned about hypoglycemia than the adult physicians in the past.

"More recent studies are showing subtle, transient effects of hypoglycemia on intellectual functioning, even in adults. A few years ago, a report showed that even after the blood sugar returns to normal, it may be up to 45 minutes before psychological testing or problem-solving skills return to normal."

"You mean that you probably shouldn't go right back to an exam or to driving after a reaction. Your ability may be impaired for quite a while?" asks Brent.

"That's what the studies seem to indicate. The neurophysiologic effects of hypoglycemia are just beginning to be understood. With tighter blood sugar management, more adults are having more reactions. Very strict blood glucose control does have some risks. In the very young children most of us think that with their brains in the rapid growth stage, it's very important to not keep them too tightly controlled, especially when they can't even tell us their symptoms."

"I was reading somewhere that it is the years after puberty that count, and the years of diabetes before puberty are not as important to the long-term complications," Lisa comments.

"There's some recent information on that point. But remember those studies are talking about complications from high blood sugar or hyperglycemia, not hypoglycemia."

Brent adds, somewhat defensively, "That shouldn't give a carte blanche to those below puberty."

"You're right, Brent. We need to control the blood sugars as best we can, but it does possibly make us a little less uptight about making sure every blood test is in the normal range. We also want to avoid putting the kids on such tight control that they have lots of lows. We must balance the information the researchers keep giving us. A middle-of-the-road approach is safest, I think."

"I remember trying so hard to keep Jeff's blood sugars within the normal range. Every time I looked at that machine and saw a high reading, like over 200, I'd get so uptight and angry. I felt very frustrated and, in a way, like a failure, because as a mother I couldn't control this thing. You know, we mothers are supposed to be able to fix everything." Lucy looks around at the other moms. They understand. But the fathers do, too. Because they would all like to make the numbers come out right. I know for sure Brent, the mathematician, would like to be able to control these numbers. It's good for him to hear that the other parents have these same frustrations.

Lucy continues, "Once I decided that these ups and downs were going to occur even if I did my darnedest, I relaxed a bit. The really high numbers still upset me, but I'm handling it better. Luckily, Jeff doesn't have too many, and his *hemoglobin A1c's* are pretty good. He's active, into everything and feeling pretty good about himself. So for that, I'm very happy."

Nancy comments, "You've done a good job with him, Lucy. He takes his diabetes so naturally. And Kyle is so supportive, too. They're both great role models for the other kids here." The other parents nod in agreement.

Lucy smiles, a bit flushed, "I guess I'm just lucky."

"Dr. MacCracken, is there any way of knowing what the blood sugars are in the middle of the night besides sticking the kids then?" asks Darryl.

"That's the only way to know for sure, but there are some clues to watch for that might give you a hint your child is having lows at night or in the very early morning. Wetting the bed can be a clue to low sugar."

Pearl comments, "I thought that happened with high sugars. Emily started to wet the bed again before we found out she had diabetes."

"Pearl, you're right. Before the diagnosis and treatment with insulin, new-onset bedwetting certainly can be caused by high blood sugar, especially when they are drinking so much. But after these children have been placed on insulin, the most common cause of bedwetting is hypoglycemia or a reaction."

"That's good to know," says Sam.

"Waking up with a headache or being slow to rise can be another clue. Of course, some kids are just not morning people."

"Some of us adults can be slow to rise too," jokes Mark, as he nudges Lisa. She gives him a little push back.

"But those mornings may be different than their usual state of arousal. Morning headaches should be looked into. We recommend, and this has been studied by several groups, that the blood sugar before bed be above 115. Children with values below this run a higher risk of having a low sugar in the night. Also, if the child wakes up with a blood sugar below 100 in the morning, they may have low sugars in the very early morning.

"Does that have something to do with the dawn phenomenon?" asks Lucy."

"The *dawn phenomenon* describes the observation that at some time in the early morning, say around 4 or 5 A.M. there is in non-diabetics an increase output of insulin that seems to be required to keep the blood sugar stable. No one knows the exact cause for increased need for insulin. Certain hormones, like growth hormone, also increase in the night. These hormones have an anti-insulin effect, and thus, more insulin is required to counteract these other hormones." I go over it again. "In folks with diabetes, no extra insulin is available from their own pancreases to counter this anti-insulin effect. Thus, the blood sugar rises. The blood sugar at 7 or 8 o'clock in the morning may be higher than it was at 4 or 5 A.M."

"So, if your blood sugar level is 80 at 7 o'clock, it might have been 50 or 60 a few hours earlier," states Brent.

"That's right. The blood sugar can rise in the morning even without the person eating. Now, again some believe that clinicians may be overemphasizing this, and that the actual rise in blood sugar is due to the waning effect of the nighttime or evening insulin injection. This certainly needs to be kept in mind. I just want you to understand the thought processes we go through when we adjust insulin dosages for the nighttime. It can be the hardest time to control things. A low *hemoglobin A1c*, a large total daily dose of insulin, and a longer duration of diabetes are also risk factors for hypoglycemia in the night."

"Becky's doctor only gets those A1c tests once a year. Do you think they should be done more frequently?" Darryl asks.

"Do you all know the test that Darryl is talking about?"

"I don't think my doctor does that. What is it?" replies Lydia.

"The hemoglobin A1c or *glycosylated hemoglobin* is a test that indicates what the average blood sugar has been for the past two to three months. Glucose binds to the hemoglobin in the red cell. Thus, the term glycosylated (glucose bound) or if it's easier you can think of it like glazing. The reds cells get glazed just like doughnuts do, and the red cell stays glazed until it's destroyed and recycled."

Sam says, "So the number of glazed red cells depends upon the amount of sugar in the blood."

"Right!"

"So, you think it should be done every three months?" asks Darryl.

"Yes, I do. I find that the kids and parents like to know what the results are, especially if there has been an improvement. Now sometimes, with very young children who are traumatized by the blood drawing and who have been running fairly consistent blood sugars and consistent past hemoglobin A1c's, I skip a time and do it every six months. With the adolescents, however, it's very important to stay right on them and give them feedback so together we can make adjustments, if necessary."

"Our doctor does the tests but never tells us the results," Darryl adds.

"I think it helps to keep your own record of the results. Pat and I send the results to the kids, and we use special stamps to give congratulations and encouragement."

"Jeff just loves to get those letters. That smiley Lion that says, 'Great Job!' really pleases him," comments Lucy.

"One last comment about glycosylated hemoglobin tests. It's important to know the normals of the laboratory where the test is done. There are different methods, and you cannot compare one to another very well. It's best to be consistent, using one lab."

After a few more questions and comments we all decide to stand up for a stretch. Suddenly Pat and all the kids come tearing down the grassy hillside. It's snack time. And for us break time. Everyone strolls up to the lodge. The trio of Peter, Kyle, and Jeff wrestle with each other all the way back up the hill. Mark and Lisa hold hands with Abigail and Little Lucy on either side.

I walk up the hill with Pat and Lucy, who is limping quite a bit. I'm sure those hard wooden seats were not the best thing for her. But she'd never complain. I say, "Lucy, I want you to know that I know it takes a lot more than luck to have such great kids as Jeff and Kyle. You are doing a marvelous job."

"Thanks," she smiles with her beautifully sensitive eyes. There are people who impress you with their sensitivity, their courage, their optimism, their special style. Lucy is one of them.

After the snack, the kids put on their play for the parents.

"Here we have a liver." Kevin points to Becky, who is holding up a sign saying, LIVER. She bows. "And over in this corner is Mr. MUSCLE." Peter does three or four jumping jacks and holds up his sign, MUSCLE. "And this is the BLOODSTREAM." Tate and Little Lucy are holding up a red, long, hollow paper pipe, a remnant from gift wrapping paper. Both are giggling as they take a bow. The audience discretely chuckles.

Pat and I produced this little skit to visually explain what exercise does to blood sugar, how exercise affects the insulin levels in non-diabetics, how the liver stores glucose as glycogen, and how the liver might be able to supply extra glucose. We were both amazed how quickly the children in our clinic understood the concepts after seeing or acting in the skit. We have incorporated it since into our camp program.

The announcer continues, "This lovely young lady is the INSULIN LEVEL." Abigail, holding her sign, does a delightful curtsy. She's such a cute kid and so interested in everything. I bet she hasn't missed a trick in this skit. "And playing the role of the STOMACH is Emily." The sign STOMACH is almost as large as Emily. But you can see her dark eyes peering above the poster board. "All the organs are in their places, so we . . . ." Kevin hesitates for a moment.

Eddy whispers, "You forgot to introduce the kid with diabetes, the kid without diabetes, and the beads."

Kevin thinks. "Oh, yes, Susan will play the non-diabetic." She smiles. "And Jeff will play the kid with diabetes." Jeff gives a little wave. And these green glass beads," he holds up a clear jar filled with little green beads, "are GLUCOSE MOLECULES."

As Cindy and Ginny give more directions, Kevin announces that they are the co-directors, and Eddy is the stage manager with Kyle assistant stage manager. So, the scene is complete. Let the show begin.

The kids do a splendid job. The several scenes flow fairly smoothly. First, we are shown what happens when a person without diabetes begins to exercise. The insulin level drops immediately. And glucose can come out of the liver to give more energy to the athlete. Then we watch the child with diabetes begin to exercise. Peter, the muscle, jumps up and down vigorously. As long as there is food in the stomach, the blood sugar will be OK. But when the athlete with diabetes exercises with an empty stomach, the blood sugar may drop. On stage we see that the insulin level may not change; it actually could rise if the extremity being exercised recently had an injection of insulin. And as Jeff falls to the floor with a low blood sugar, we are shown that the glucose cannot come out of the liver for an energy source as long as too much insulin is around.

The parents are enjoying the show and learning about exercise and diabetes at the same time. The final scene illustrates why a child with diabetes who already has a high blood sugar can make things worse by exercising. Jeff, the kid with diabetes, starts to exercise. The blood stream is filled with green beads (glucose molecules). With lack of insulin (Abigail is lying on the floor, showing a low level of insulin), no glucose can go into the muscle. (Peter, the muscle, acts like he is starving.) Because the level of insulin is very low, the liver can dump more glucose into the bloodstream. (Becky, the liver, puts more green beads into the red tube,) The system is ineffective without the proper level of insulin; too much can cause low blood sugar, and too little can cause higher blood sugar.

The children take a bow. The audience applauds. Then Pat has the kids list some exercise tips: Remember to eat your meal or snack before you exercise, keep a quick source of energy easily available, and if you have ketones or a very high blood sugar, don't exercise. Pat hands out a sheet listing the factors that affect the hypoglycemic response to exercise, as well as suggestions for preventing the problem.

"Now that makes sense. Why didn't Susan's doctor just do a little skit for us," says Brent. The other parents laugh.

"Well, I don't know. But we think the skit helps illustrate these important points about exercise. Somehow if you understand a little bit about the chemical changes in the body, it's easier to remember the rules about exercising."

"How many calories are required?" Brent asks.

Pat comments, "We recommend 15 grams of carbohydrate for each half an hour of mild exercise and twice that for each half hour of strenuous exercise."

"Would playing little league baseball be mild, moderate, or strenuous exercise?"

"I suppose that depends if you're the pitcher, catcher, or an outfielder who never gets the ball," Eddy comments. As he says that, Tate winds up and throws an imaginary ball, which Peter pretends to catch.

Outside the window I notice a large, shiny new maroon pick-up truck going around the circle slowly. Its driver parks by the No

Parking sign and gets out. He's a big, muscular man with a white T-shirt and blue overalls. The lobster traps in the back of his truck give away his identity. He must be Lou, arriving for the afternoon outing to the Bangor Mall. Lydia sees him too. She leaves the room.

"Let's see, only Brent, Marjorie, Tate, and Susan will be gone for supper, is that right?" Pat asks.

"Nancy and I will be back after supper, too" says Darryl. Great, that means they've taken my suggestion to have a quiet dinner together.

"Eddy, I'll be back for the baseball game," says Tate. Both Tate and Eddy have their baseball caps on backwards.

Most folks head off to gather their things and pick up a sack lunch before departure. Lydia brings Lou in to meet Pat and me. He's a very large man. I'd guess six feet four inches, at least, and maybe 250 pounds. I wonder how many pounds of lobster he pushes around every day. We shake hands. His feels like a baseball mitt. Lou's clean shaven and looks younger than Lydia. Both seem happy to see each other. She doesn't look so large, as she stands next to him. Cindy stands behind them. I don't see Kevin.

"I'm glad you could come. Lydia has told us about you," says Pat.

"This is quite a place you've got here," Lou comments.

"Thanks, we love it. It has a special atmosphere. Will you be back for supper?" Pat inquires.

"I don't know. I probably will have to get back. Got traps to check."

"Well, hope you have a good time at the Mall."

"Is that where we're going?" he jokes, giving Lydia a small squeeze. She smiles like a little kid on Christmas morning.

"I told you that's what we wanted to do," she adds, nudging him.

Cindy's enjoying Lydia and Lou teasing each other. I don't imagine Lydia gets many positive strokes from others.

"Well, have a good time. It ought to take you about 40 minutes to get there." I say. I wonder where Kevin is. Does he plan on boycotting this trip? I hope not.

Nancy and Darryl are the first to take off. "Have fun, and don't worry about Becky. She'll have a good time with us in Ellsworth and at Fort Knox," I say.

"Will do," says Darryl. He looks genuinely eager to get away with Nancy. I can't quite read her expression. She's probably worried about Becky, but knows that's silly.

As they drive off, I notice Becky standing in the doorway. She has the same expression on her face. Is she worried, too? Cindy speaks briefly to Becky and then joins Lydia, Lou, and Kevin over at the pickup. Somehow, all four of those large people fit into the front seat. Becky, Pat, and I wave good-bye and the truck leaves a dust cloud behind.

The Blue Hill group pulls away. Tate waves his baseball hat out the window. I hope Brent and Marjorie enjoy their reminiscent reconnoitering with kids. And I hope Susan gets through the day without a reaction.

The rest of us wait around for the lunch bell, which invites us to a pleasant outdoor picnic. Our Camp Kee-to-Kin family has definitely grown smaller. We fit around two picnic tables.

CHAPTER 9

In Search
of the Big Picture

After lunch we take off for Ellsworth. Ginny and Becky sit in the back, and Eddy grabs the front passenger seat. As we head on down the road, my radio comes on playing some fine classical music.

"Come on, Doc, let's go for something a bit more lively," Eddy quips.

"OK, you be the tunes man, and if there's nothing good on the radio, you can always check out my tapes," I suggest.

After a few station changes, Eddy asks, "Hey, Doc, where are your tapes?"

"They're tucked under your seat in an orange box. It's quite a varied collection. I should warn you."

"This should be interesting." He smiles as he reaches under the seat.

"The Mamas and the Papas! Dr. MacCracken, you really are over the hill." And he laughs. I can laugh at that, too. I happen to love their music but usually have to play it when I'm all by myself because neither my husband nor my kids can stand it.

"Eddy, turn up the radio," Becky requests. I suggest that instead of turning up this awful hard rock, he simply adjust the back speakers.

"Hey, you guys want to listen to some Navajo music?" Eddy jests. He's found my special tape. It's beautiful to those of us who have lived in the Southwest and have been associated with Navajo. But otherwise those chants would sound very unreal, almost surrealistic.

"You'd find the music very strange. I lived on the Navajo Indian reservation for two years, so it kind of takes me back."

Eddy asks me about the reservation. He has always wanted to get off the East Coast and explore the USA. I encourage him to try it. There's nothing like it to open your eyes, to expand your mind, to encounter new people. He tells me about the article he read about this girl with diabetes who rode her bicycle all around the country. Maybe he would make it a motorcycle, instead. I knew the girl who did that trip. And she surely grew from the experience. It would be great for Eddy to explore, too. And certainly, there's no need for his diabetes to hold him down.

Ginny and Becky lean forward, trying to listen to our conversation. I'm pleased that Becky hears our discussion of exploration and adventure. Ginny realizes diabetes doesn't have to tie you down. She went to on an Outward Bound program on Hurricane Island last summer.

I reach for the radio and turn down the volume. "Ginny, would you do that Outward Bound program again?" I know the answer, and I know she knows I know the answer, but I also know she knows why I ask.

"It was the most awesome time I've ever had. A real challenge, and the staff let us make all the decisions ourselves. And we had to live with the consequences. Once, we almost got caught by the tide before we could land, but a few fast thinking kids saved us. The day alone on the island was incredible. I was a little scared, but it was good for me."

"Were you all alone, really?" Becky is shocked.

"Well, this other girl and I were on the island, but we weren't supposed to meet in the center until evening. And we didn't either. I enjoyed my solitude. Some of the other kids joined each other as soon as they were dropped off, but Laura and I followed the rules and met about sunset time to build a lean-to. What a fabulous night! We saw the Northern Lights."

"So, you'd obviously recommend that experience?" I ask.

"Sure, but I'm going to sign up for the western version, maybe next summer. I feel safe on the sea now, but not on a mountain top. I want to learn to repel. That would be awesome!"

"I think we can pass up the bagpipe music." Eddy is still looking through my fabulous wealth of diverse recordings. "This 'Mom's Super Tape' looks interesting. What's on it?"

"Oh, you'll like that. My son made it for me. He chose all the popular groups who aren't too loud or heavy (metal I mean) and put them together. It's got Bobby McFerrin's 'Don't Worry, Be Happy' and some Paul Simon and the Black Mombazo Band, Eagles, and Grateful Dead. There's even some Beatles on there."

"That sounds good. I'll try it." He flips the tape into my sound system. Immediately the whistling of Bobby McFerrin comes on, and then the words, "Here's a little song I wrote, You might want to sing it note for note, Don't worry, Be happy. ... " Such a spunky jingle. The song continues, "In every life we have some trouble. When you worry you make it double, Don't Worry, Be Happy ... " In the rearview mirror I spot Becky.

If the whole world could be happy—what a Pollyannic philosophy. I guess it's the worry that's the unnecessary part. Mark Twain once said something like "We worry about so many things that never come true." Worrying doesn't help. It seems like these days even the kids have to worry. They are so battered by adult concerns like drugs, AIDS, nuclear war, starvation, the homeless. We include the children so early in our worries. I think we need to give the children time to play. And then there's diabetes. The worries of all that. The responsibilities. My mind drifts.

"Dr. MacCracken . . . Dr. MacCracken." It's Becky. "I have to go to the bathroom."

I'm snapped out of my private thoughts. "Oh, sure, we'll stop up ahead at the Exxon station."

We stop. I fill up with gas, and Eddy checks the oil for me while Ginny and Becky visit the ladies room. Ginny has definitely taken on Becky. Earlier Ginny told me she thinks she can help Becky and was quite delighted to have her come with us. She already thinks Becky is getting the bigger picture—like the entire world isn't going to wait on her, and her diabetes is not her parents' fault, and her mother needs to stop worrying about her so much and do something for herself. And even more, that she's a lot luckier than some kids, like Cindy, for example. Ginny feels a change in Becky. I can't really tell. She hasn't exactly warmed up to me.

Some kids gravitate towards me, while others don't. This year Susan likes to hang around me. Maybe she's psychic and knows I'm the answer to her reactions. Well, that's not quite fair, but I'm determined to help her feel better. She shouldn't have so many lows. Hopefully, she's having fun in Blue Hill. With some extra snacks, she ought to make it up that mountain just fine. Tate'll probably run up all the way. I picture Marjorie and Brent strolling up the path, perhaps yearning for those carefree days. Four children, college tuitions, research grant applications, diabetes, sexually active teenagers, worries, worries. Problems parents face today. What does the song say, "Don't Worry, Be Happy."

My thoughts continue. Susan and Emily are special kids to me this year. Emily is coming out of her shell. She wants to learn, and because of that, Sam does, too. By decreasing his intermediate insulin, he ought to be feeling better this afternoon, not craving the whole refrigerator, like Pearl said.

"You need a quart of oil," Eddy calls from the other side of the hood. He holds up the stick to show me.

"Fine, I use 10W/40."

With full tanks of gas and oil and with empty bladders, we take off for our destination, Ellsworth, Maine, and the new L.L.Bean outlet store. The music blares on. I drive along, appreciating the purple and pink lupine by the roadside. Sunlight comes and goes as more clouds gather.

For about an hour, we wander around the outlet clothing and

sports stores. The kids spend most of their time in the drug store checking out post cards and other knickknacks. By 2:30, I start to think of heading back. We should have a snack first before meeting Pat at Fort Knox around 3:15. These kids will need one, especially with hiking at Fort Knox.

Eddy feels pretty hungry and gets two plain donuts. Ginny buys an apple-cinnamon granola bar. Becky takes a long time to choose. If none of us were here, she might make a different choice, but in the end, she buys a granola bar, too. I get some beef jerky for myself and two spare granola bars for the hike.

We pull into the Fort Knox parking lot as Pat arrives in her van. Perfect timing. Jeff, Kyle, and Peter leap out of the van followed by Big Lucy, Mark, Sam, and Emily. Pearl stayed at camp for a nap, and Lisa and her two girls, Abigail and Little Lucy, wanted more time on the beach. So, we have a total of 12. I pay the group rate, and we head toward the fort.

"How many flashlights have we got?" I ask.

Pat replies, "Mark, Sam, and I have flashlights. Jeff has his own."

"Let's try to stay in a group. We don't need anyone getting lost in those tunnels," I add. I've only done this tour twice, but Pat comes every year. She can lead. Emily grabs my hand, as we descend the first stone stairway.

It's an impressive fort, built in 1846 on the cliffs overlooking the Penobscot River, just above the town of Bucksport. Huge cannons peer through the small openings in the thick stone walls. It's the closest thing to a medieval castle that Maine has to offer. Jeff, Kyle, and Peter hide behind large pillars and fire their imaginary guns.

We enter the lower fortress. Already we are separated. It's hopeless to keep this group together. Sam leads our group with his light. I'm behind him with Emily. Ginny and Becky are behind me. All we can see is a narrow beam of light at the end of the walk. The chill of the damp granite stone walls contrasts to the warm sun just outside. I hear another group in the next corridor. It must be the boys, for the hooting and pretend gunfire are recognizable. Mark or Eddy must be with them.

"Two steps up," says Sam, warning us about a brief staircase.

Continuing down a long corridor, we come out into the kitchen and mess hall. Big ovens are built into the walls. The other group of Mark, Eddy, and the three boys enter the kitchen from another hall. That's ten of us. Who are we missing? Pat and Lucy must be in another tunnel. Jeff asks if we have seen his mother. No one has, but I tell him she must be with Pat, who has a flashlight and knows the tunnels. In the corner of the kitchen is a circular staircase leading up to the roof for a good view of the river. All ten of us climb up. I hope Pat and Lucy are okay.

After walking around we descend the same staircase back into the kitchen. Still no sign of Pat and Lucy. As the others walk out onto the grassy inner courtyard, I whistle my standard signal, which I know Pat would recognize. No response. Damn, where could they be?

There are endless crisscrossing passages back in there. I instruct Mark and Eddy to keep an eye on everyone else. "Just let them look in the other rooms off the courtyard. Don't leave this area." I explain to Emily that her dad and I are going to look for Pat and Lucy, and she needs to stay here with Ginny and Becky.

"Come back soon," she whispers.

"We'll be right back, Em." Her father reassures her.

Jeff insists that he come with us to find his mom and Pat. He looks so worried that I agree. "Jeff, don't worry, Pat knows these tunnels. Besides, even if they took the wrong turn, there is really no danger."

"But she could fall on that slippery floor." He's an astute seven year old who has perhaps seen his mom fall before. "My dad tells her to take it easy, but she won't listen. I should have told her to stay in the van."

"Hey, Jeff, she's going to be fine. Let's go," Sam says.

With two flashlights, Jeff and I go down the passageway that I came in through. Sam goes down the other tunnel. We plan to give a call if we find anything. I also whistle every few seconds to alert Sam to our location and to connect with Pat. In between one of my whistle I hear a distant call. It's not Sam; it must be Pat or Lucy. We proceed down the tunnel, and the voice gets louder. Then I see Pat.

"Lucy fell on some steps. She's okay but bruised her hip and knee. I think we'll have to carry her out." Just then we see Sam's flashlight across the tunnel. He's found a connecting hallway.

"Lucy fell and will need to be carried out. Should we get some others?" I ask him.

"Where is she? I think I can carry her." Sam, Jeff, and I proceed down the tunnel. Pat goes to tell the others what has happened, and we agree to all meet at the back entrance. We find Lucy calmly sitting with Pat's flashlight. Jeff gives his mom a hug.

"Oh, Jeffrey, I'm all right. What a stupid thing for me to do. I just misjudged those little steps. I should've been more careful, I guess. My knee and hip don't want to move."

"Are you in a lot of pain?" I ask.

"No, not really."

Sam says, "We'll get you out of here in no time." He leans over and lifts Lucy gently into the air. "You weigh less than two sacks of potatoes." And she probably does, too. Big Lucy's probably not much more than 95 pounds. But to Jeffrey, Sam is a giant, a mighty strong hero at that. With his red and black checked shirt he even looks like Paul Bunyan. Jeff and I light the way, as Sam deftly carries Lucy.

Pat has everyone gathered at the back entrance and has brought the van around. Sam places Lucy in the front seat. Kyle comes over to check on his mom. She kisses him on the forehead. Her knee is bruised and swollen. She flexes her hip. I note no point tenderness. Doubt that it's broken, just badly bruised. We'll go back to camp and reevaluate. Steve, her husband, is coming for the campfire, and there'll be time to see if she needs to go to Bangor for x-rays.

Heavy dark clouds drift in from the north as we pull out of the parking lot. Storm tonight, I'd guess.

C H A P T E R   10

Ketones and Overtones

Back at Hersey Retreat, Heather has returned and relates that all is quiet at the hospital. We always hope no major problems arise while all three of us are here. On her drive back she kept just ahead of a thunderstorm.

Lucy awaits the arrival of Steve. Hoping their dad will arrive soon, her sons sit anxiously by the window. Storm clouds blacken the sky towards Bangor. A flash of lightning lights the northwest sky. No thunder follows. It's still quite a bit north. Pat and I discuss the plans for the camp fire. There's no chance of a calm fire on the beach. We activate plan B. In the attic, we cut out some orange and yellow flames from construction paper. The campfire will be held in the game room. We'll still sing our songs, and joke around.

Both of us feel bad about Lucy's fall. We never should have taken her to Fort Knox. But she insisted. We recall other campers in past years who have had medical problems. It seems like just last year when all these people were with us. Yet, they have been here over the past nine years. They've each added an extra touch to the week, giving, somehow, a more universal outlook, so we don't become completely focused on the problems of diabetes. We are reminded of other illnesses. And lessons have been learned—of patience, of inner strength, and of the mature sense of self, whatever the burden.

One father brought his daughter to camp. He had hemophilia and his joints were damaged from years of bumps, bruises, and bleeding. He had known the pain of disease, the necessity of his injections to prevent the bleeding. He carried on, trying to help his daughter who now faced injections of a different nature. I'll always remember him. A few years later he died from complications of his disease. But for me, his courage lives on.

We had a mother with multiple sclerosis whose grand mal seizure at camp added to our medical trials of the week. But as Pat and I think about this episode, we laugh. This mother had warned us that she might have a seizure. She told us that after her seizures, she's usually quite confused, and what we need to do is tell her who she is and where she is, over and over. I made a mental note of that.

Well, Alice had her seizure in the downstairs bathroom one morning. It lasted a few minutes. Pat and I squeezed into the small bathroom and shut the door, so the other campers would not be upset. Just imagine a rather large lady lying on the floor half way in the shower stall, and two of us trying to be sure she didn't bit her tongue or aspirate.

She stopped seizing, opened her eyes, and stared blankly at me. I remembered and started to say, "You're Alice Hope, and you're at Hersey Retreat, You're Alice Hope, and you are at Hersey Retreat." Again, as I squeezed her hand, "You're Alice Hope, and you're at Hersey Retreat."

She spoke, "I know who I am. But who the hell are you?" Pat and I burst out laughing. Comic relief, I guess you could say. Well, I told her who I was. She recovered slowly from the seizure. That was a tough week. But Pat and I will never forget that line—"Who the hell are you?"

Ginny comes up to remind us it's blood testing time. We've lost track of time in our reminiscing. Most of the kids have started on their own and have even recorded their readings on their charts. Coming downstairs, we see Becky who, to our great surprise and pleasure, is helping Emily put the drop of blood onto the meter. Pearl stands to the side.

"I didn't cry at all." Emily's big brown eyes are wide open. "Becky helped me. She's good." I suppose she means Becky didn't hurt her with the pricker. Pat puts her arm around Becky's shoulder and says, "Great job, Emily! That's a big step." Pearl grins. I wish that Darryl and Nancy could see their daughter at this moment. But they're still out, having a good time, I hope.

Jeff taps Pat on the elbow. "Pat, before my dad gets here, I want to give my own injection." I know Jeff has made this a goal. He wants to help with his own diabetes because his mother's fingers are quite stiff. And after Lucy's fall this afternoon, he may be even more determined.

"Do you know your dose?" Pat asks.

"Yep, and I have the bottles here, too. My blood sugar was 109."

"Great, let's do it," Pat replies. Carefully and methodically, Jeff goes through the steps of drawing up the two types of insulin, just as Pat has taught him. With each step, he looks for Pat's approval. "You're doing just fine." Then he puts down the syringe and wipes his thigh with an alcohol swab.

As he lets that dry, he loads his Inject-Ease®, a neat little gadget for the younger kids or anyone who just can't bring themselves to plunge the needle into the skin. Jeff pinches the skin of his thigh and places the Inject-Ease on site. He looks at Pat and the group that has gathered. Emily, Abigail, Kyle, and Sam are all watching. Jeff's mom is within ear shot.

"You can do it," encourages his brother.

"Just push the button," Pat instructs.

"Click." His hand is steady. He makes no wince, as he slowly injects the insulin by pushing the syringe's plunger. Pleased, he pulls out the needle, and kids applaud. That's a big step for this seven year old! Jeff runs over to his mother and gets a big hug. Kyle joins them, as they continue to watch for Steve.

I notice Sam recording his blood sugar on his chart, which Pat only put up this morning. If we're going to be adjusting his insulin, we've got to know its effect. He doesn't seem to mind writing it down. His energy level seemed fine this afternoon, as he carried Lucy from the tunnel. Sam comes over, and we discuss his dosage for this evening. He says he felt fine all afternoon. He's a little hungry now, but not like usual.

We pick a dosage that is about one-third of his total daily dose. That's sort of a starting point we use, two-thirds of the total dose in the morning and one-third at night. I suggest equal amounts of regular (short-acting) and *NPH (intermediate-acting)* insulin for the evening dose, another rule of thumb. Of course, those of us in this field realize this is just a starting point and with each individual case, we must make minor adjustments. But it's a start. Emily watches her dad draw up his insulin. She doesn't miss a trick. Who knows. We may just have her give herself a shot before the end of the week.

"Here comes Dad!" Jeff runs to meet his father. Kyle's close behind. Wearing a wet jacket Steve enters, his boys on either side. Steve gives his wife a kiss.

"You're soaked," she comments.

"Yeah, the downpour got me just as I got off work." Steve works at the James River Company in Old Town. "I think I'm just ahead of the storm now. It'll be coming soon, and there's wind with it."

"Everyone, this is Steve, Kyle and Jeff's dad, as I'm sure you can tell. He'll be with us this evening, so introduce yourselves at supper or after. Now, we better get to supper. Bring your raincoats.

Eddy, would you grab a few umbrellas from that carton?" The wind increases and the sky darkens as we hurry over to the French house. Lightning and thunder soon fill the sky. The thunder scares Little Lucy. We all count after each streak of lightning. Sitting there on the high bluff, the main lodge is very exposed to the high winds. But the French House is cozy and warm.

Pat stands to give announcements. "I guess we can't have the campfire on the beach, but we'll have it in the game room with special effects. Everyone be thinking of your favorite songs, and we'll sing all night. Let's hope Cindy and Nancy get back in time to help the women's section. Dr. MacCracken and I need lots of singers. Mark promises to tell a Downeast Maine story or two."

The lights flicker.

Pat continues, "And tonight we have two special announcements. Trumpet, please."

I blare out in horny fashion, "Ta, ta ,ta, ta, . . . ta, taaaa."

"Before supper, Jeff, with precision and excellence, drew up and injected his insulin all by himself." She claps, and everyone joins in. Steve pats his son on the back, as Jeff blushes just a bit. His mother grins from ear to ear. "And a very young lady this evening without any tears or fuss did her blood test with just a little assistance from Becky. Emily, congratulations!"

Again we all applaud, but I think her grandmother and father clap the hardest. Becky, sitting next to Emily, holds up Emily's hand, as a referee would the triumphant boxer. With her newly adopted younger sister, Becky glows for the first time.

Once more the lights blink on and off. Just in case, I locate the flashlight that Laurie, our cook, always keeps handy above the kitchen table. She's busy lighting some candles and placing them at strategic locations. She reminds me that this point of land is well-known for its power outages. And, as if she were psychic, the lights flicker again and then go out.

The candlelight is sufficient for us to complete our scrumptious dessert. You can't even tell it's made with artificial sweetener. The kids devour their helpings. Emily, who is across from me at the table, sums it all up, "Yummy," she says. The dishwashers, who luckily are not electric, do a stellar job in the limited lighting. We all wait to go back together, assuming the main lodge will be dark. The thunder rolls in the distance now. Rain hits the windowpanes, but the wind lessens.

Sam volunteers to start a fire in the fireplace for light and heat. With flashlight in hand, I escort the campers to their rooms where they locate their own flashlights. "Flashlight" is on the list of recommended supplies to bring.

As I come downstairs, Emily, with chocolate pudding still on her nose, asks me to take her to her room to find Inky, her black stuffed rabbit. She says she's afraid he'll be scared in the dark. And maybe Emily is just a little scared without him. Sam and Pearl are still working on the fire. We walk upstairs, holding hands.

I haven't been in this room for awhile. It used to be the one that Pat and I slept in. Two large windows face the water. Though it's dark in the lodge, it is a little lighter outside, and I see a field of whipped white caps. Glad I'm not at sea. I shine my flashlight on the double bed. A country quilt neatly covers the bed, and a bathrobe and nightgown are in a tidy pile. No Inky here. Both bunkbeds are made with military precision. Sam's flashlight is on his bed. Still, no Inky. Emily points to the dresser. My light shines on the dresser top. It's hard to believe I'm still at Hersey Retreat, where most rooms are stark and bare. A picture frame catches my eye. In the photo three boys stand together, holding their fishing poles. The boy with the red hair must be Sam, and probably the other boys are his brothers.

Another smaller photo shows Pearl standing with a gentle looking man, probably Ollie. Near the bed, there's a Bible. Something orange reflects my light. Out of curiosity, I look closer. The profile of a man's head is stamped in relief on a piece of thin copper, and below are the words: Prayer of St. Francis of Assisi. I've heard these words before. "Lord, make me an instrument of your Peace, Where there is . . . ."

Emily pulls on my arm. "Maybe, Inky's under the bed." She takes my flashlight and bends down. "There you are, Inky. Me and Dr. MacQuacken was looking for you. Are you OK?" She hugs her special rabbit. I grab Sam's flashlight off his bed, and we three head back downstairs.

The fire's roaring now, and firelight throws large shadows on the walls as the campers move around. Pat and Eddy arrange the chairs in a big semi-circle around the fireplace. Now that we have a real fire, there's no need for our artificial flames. We'll save those yellow and orange flames for next year, or the next.

"Okay, everybody pick a partner. We're going to teach you a song with action." Pat pulls me into the middle of the semi-circle. The fire crackles. She and I have a great time demonstrating this song, and the campers practice and get faster and faster. We all laugh. Nancy and Darryl walk in. Both are drenched, but appear oblivious to that. They tell us that the power is out all along the coast. It must be a major outage.

"Well, that means it may get fixed sooner, than later, if a large area is involved," I add. "Get some dry clothes on, and come join us. We're getting warmed up for a sing-a-long."

Becky gives them her flashlight. "We'll be right down," Darryl says, as he and Nancy head upstairs.

Their return reminds me of the other missing flocks. The Bangor Mall crew hasn't been seen yet, nor the Blue Hill contingent. I assume they're waiting for the storm to pass. Driving on these back roads in heavy rain is treacherous. But they should all be back soon. With no baseball game, Tate probably wasn't pushing as hard for an early return.

"Should we start out with something easy, like 'Old MacDonald'?"

"Yeah!" says Little Lucy. And we all do a good rendition of that old standby. We have cows, pigs, ducks, horses, dogs, and rabbits. Next we sing a shortened version of "There's a Hole in the Bucket" and then a lengthy rendition of "I Know An Old Lady Who Swallowed a Fly." Mark and Eddy request "Down by the Old Mill Stream." I think these men like to croon. With Brent and Darryl, they might have enough for a barbershop quartet.

The fire reminds me of an old Indian chant I learned years ago. "Here's a new one for you," I say and proceed to teach the main chant and a background chant that sound almost like drums beating. The campers catch on fast.

Headlights shine through the big lodge windows. A second vehicle follows. The Booth family, all decked out in yellow rain slickers, returns from Blue Hill. Tate's yellow rain hat almost covers his entire face. We can just see his mouth and nose. "You got no lights, either? Boy, it's weird out there with no lights."

We hold up on songs for awhile, as Kevin, Cindy, and Lydia walk in. Even in the firelight, it's easy to notice Kevin's brand new fluorescent trimmed Nike Air high tops. Lou must have bought them. I wonder if this will be the way to Kevin's heart. Lydia carries a bag marked 'Sears.' Cindy's bag is from 'The Gap,' a favorite clothing store for teenagers. Christmas six months early.

"Now that everyone's back safely, Mark's going to tell us one of his Maine stories. Let's pull up that bench for the new arrivals," Pat instructs.

Mark's rich voice and sparkling eyes add greatly to the humor of his tales, not to mention his fairly authentic Maine accent. The whole group is well entertained. Obviously, from their hearty laughs, Nancy and Darryl have never heard these stories before. Mark stops and promises one or two more at the talent show. As he receives a round of applause, the lights go on.

"Great timing," says Pat. "Let's do our blood sugars, have a snack, and then we can finish off with a few peaceful songs."

I overhear Tate telling Kyle about his mountain climb. Brent watches Susan do her test. Marjorie looks content, but tired. The mountain climb was more than she remembered. But Blue Hill is as lovely as ever. Very little has changed in the past 30 years—a few new stores—but the cozy Maine coastal town feeling remains. They dream of retiring there.

"It's 110," Brent says. "Susan, that's great."

"And climbing the mountain was fun, too," Susan replies.

Susan's pink face is a great improvement over her pale complexion of yesterday. I bet she feels better, too. Less insulin has made a difference.

Kevin's blood sugar is over 300 tonight. I notice that his lunch reading was also over 300. I suspect his prelunch value was due to anxiety over Lou's coming and this reading is due to some "dietary indiscretion" at the Bangor Mall.

But with two elevated sugars, it's wise to check for urinary ketones, which can appear when high blood sugars occur. His breath has a fruity smell, like ketones that are excreted in urine and in the lung when fat is breaking down. *Ketones* smell like nail polish remover, acetone. I send Kevin to the bathroom to check a urine sample for ketones. He returns with the plastic dipstick. The bluish-purple color on the dipstick indicates moderate ketones.

Lydia comes over, "Did he tell you he forgot his insulin?"

"Mom, I thought you had it. And besides, you told me we'd be back for supper. It ain't my fault," Kevin responds, defensively.

"Yeah, but haven't I told you before to bring your supplies just in case." She's angry. "It's almost like you did it on purpose, just to get me upset and Lou mad. And he went and bought you those new expensive sneakers, too."

"Mom, I'm sorry, I really didn't do it on purpose." She looks at him in some disbelief, but makes no further comment. Kevin's eyes are on the floor, as he continues to hold the ketone strip in his hand.

"Kevin, did you eat a good supper at the Mall?"

Without looking up, Kevin admits, "We ate Kentucky Fried Chicken with coleslaw. And, I had a diet soda."

"How many pieces?" Lydia interrogates.

"Two or three."

"More like four or five." Lydia replies.

"Well, I didn't eat no biscuits or gravy like you did."

"That's only 'cuz Lou took them away from you."

"OK," I interrupt. "We need to do something about Kevin's ketones, and we need to get some insulin into him before it gets any later." Giving his NPH or intermediate acting insulin now is no problem. It's a common practice to give a third shot before bed. But the regular insulin, which is supposed to be given before the meal, can sometimes cause problems in the night if not given before a meal. But with a blood sugar of 300 and moderate ketones, Kevin's body needs regular insulin and will be able to tolerate a pretty good dose. If we don't get this under control, Kevin will just become more ketotic over the night.

I recommend a few units more than his usual NPH dose, as well as a few units less than his usual dose of regular. Later, around midnight, his mother will help him check his blood sugar and urine ketones. If his blood sugar is still over 300 and his ketones are still moderate or large, they should send Ginny to get me. But if both blood sugar and ketones are less, he'll probably be fine. Kevin takes his shot and returns to the game room.

While I deal with Lydia and Kevin, Pat checks all the other evening blood sugars. The group gathers back in the game room for a few bedtime songs. Tate, the usual source of boundless energy, sits on his mother's lap, almost asleep. Marjorie eyes are closed; perhaps she's dreaming of her white Cape with dark green shutters overlooking Blue Hill Bay. Emily and Inky sit on Pat's knee. "Let's turn the lights down," Pat suggests. We sing "He's Got the Whole World in His Hands" and "Amazing Grace." Most everyone sings along. Nancy and Cindy especially enjoy harmonizing. We end with "Taps." The fire crackles and dances. It's quiet. Emily and Little Lucy are asleep, as are Tate and Marjorie.

Finally, each family gathers and heads upstairs. Steve assists Lucy up the steps. Her knee is less swollen. He'll spend the night and leave bright and early for the mill. I remind Lydia to send for me if there's any problem with Kevin's tests. She tells me she probably shouldn't have gotten so angry. They actually all had a good time until just before supper. Lou and Kevin joked around quite a bit. "It's going to work out, Lydia, if you all just keep trying." I pat her on the back, as she heads upstairs.

Heather checks on refrigerator food supplies, and Pat finishes talking with Nancy and Darryl. The three older girls, Ginny, Becky, and Cindy, quietly talk in front of the fading embers. They plan to work on their act for the talent show. I strongly encourage them, for so far only three acts have signed up. "Don't worry about acts, Dr. MacCracken, we'll have enough," Ginny says, confidently. She must know something I don't.

"Good night, ladies," Sam says, as we leave. Alone outside, he appears to be enjoying his evening cigarette.

"Good night, Sam, and thanks again for your help with Lucy."

"No, problem, Doc. See you in the morning." I'm so glad he stayed.

Dodging the puddles along the road, we walk back to the cabin. Heather asks, "Do you think Kevin will be okay?"

"I hope so."

Heather adds, "That family sure has its problems. Lydia just can't see how hard it is for Kevin to watch what he eats while she's chowing down on gravy and biscuits."

"Sure are nice sneakers Kevin got. Do you think Lou bought them?"

"Yeah, Lydia said so. Cindy and Lydia had packages, too."

"Lobstering must be good this year," Heather comments.

We all collapse on the sofa. Two days to go. "Look, you guys, we've got work to do tonight. We haven't started to write the words to our annual Camp Kee-to-Kin song, and I haven't practiced playing my recorder since last year. Heather, I brought an extra for you, so all three of us can play our round." Pat's always thinking and keeping us on track.

"What were those songs that go together, anyway? I can never remember. . .let's see, I know it's 'Row, Row, Row, your Boat.'

"And 'Oueluette' and . . .'Three Blind Mice'."

"No, that's too long, but it's something like that. Oh, yes, it's 'Three Jolly Fishermen'."

"That's it," shouts Pat. She immediately starts to play 'Three Jolly Fishermen' as she passes the extra recorder to Heather. I begin with "Row, Row," and soon we are all practicing these three songs. Several years ago Pat and I discovered that these songs can be played simultaneously, and they will end at the same time, and the notes are harmonious.

We alternate the tunes. With Heather participating, we'll all play each song once, and we should end up at the same time. This will be no easy task. As soon as you start listening to the other players, you drift into their song. The challenge is to play together, but hold your own. So, for the next 15 minutes or so, we practice. I find that toe tapping helps, while Pat moves her head to the beat, and Heather just bursts out laughing when she misses her notes. Can't deny it takes your mind off everything else.

We break for some cheese and crackers and diet Pepsi, which Heather brought from Bangor. We munch. Pat recounts her conversation with Nancy and Darryl. "They had a great time, according to both of them. The afternoon was beautiful in Camden, and they saw the Old Windjammer Schooners moored there. They even took a dry dock tour of the 'Mary Day,' one of the old schooners. Catch this, they've decided to sign up for a week's cruise next summer. Darryl said it's time they take another honeymoon. They've never left Becky for a week. They said she'll be 13 soon and can stay with her grandmother."

"Boy, that's quite a decision. Amazing what a blue sky day in Camden, Maine can do for you."

"MacCracken, you planned this—and it actually worked," Heather comments.

"Yeah, I'll take all the credit."

"That just may be the miracle they were looking for."

"Maybe."

"Okay, we need to get back to songwriting. I have the old words from last year. We should be able to alter them and use the same ending." Pat hands out the old version from last year, and I get the one from the year before. I can't remember what year we started this song, but I think it was the second or third season."

"We'll start out, 'Oh, it's the tenth great year that we have been, right down here at Kee-to-Kin, with friends from away and'.... By eleven we've about perfected the song. We'll work on the entrance and exit dance routine tomorrow night. So far, we have the recorder songs and our annual Andrew Sisters version of "Side by Side."

"I'd love to write another song. What tune could we use?" I ask. As I reach for another cracker, Heather absentmindedly hums the Indian chant song. Pat picks up the beat, and Heather sings out, "Insulin, Insulin, Insulin, Insulin," to the chant. I pick up two pieces of wood near the stove and bang them together to the beat. 'Lower your sugar, Lower your sugar.' And we've got it. A new version of an old chant. For another hour we create the words and the dance to go with it. This'll kill them. Heather will be the hit of the talent show. A gem of a skit. We'll pick out the costumes tomorrow.

At midnight, we realize if we don't get to bed, tomorrow will be here too soon. But we are, as some say, pumped. We laugh 'til we cry with hysterics. Chief Somoygi and The Rebounds will be ready.

Humming myself to sleep, I assume Kevin is fine. It's just after midnight, and no one has come for us.

Getting
Intimate
with Insulin

By Thursday morning Pat, Heather, and I always wonder if we've taught enough or if there's enough time left to teach all the things we should. This morning the educational topics will be insulin, its timing, and injection techniques. Basic important information.

When Pat rings the bell for the morning session, the adults slowly start to assemble. Only five balls remain on the pool table. Kevin and Peter are reluctant to stop, but I assure them that they can finish their game later. Tate and Abigail gladly give up their game of ping-pong, for them mostly a hit-and-chase-the-ball game. An extra ring of the bell brings the rest of the kids in from outside or upstairs.

"What are we doing now?" asks Susan, as she grabs my hand.

"We're going to have a little fun," I reply. I smile and wink at Pat.

Pat hands out a bottle of insulin to each child.

"Now, the label tells us lots of things about insulin. Who can tell me the type of insulin in your bottle?"

Susan raises her hand, and Peter waves his hand madly, yelling

"I know, I know!" Tate shouts out, "Lilly, Lilly!"

"Actually, Lilly is the Company name or brand name, Tate. We'll talk about that in a minute. Now, what type of insulin? Susan, what do you think?"

"Pork," she said proudly.

"That's right. Who has another type?"

"Mine says 'human.' Eek, is it from a human?" says Abigail.

"Pork comes from pigs and varies from human insulin only by one amino acid, a small part of the protein. But the human insulin in your bottle is not from humans. It's made by bioengineering." I say that slowly. "The drug companies have scientists, bioengineers, who take bacteria called E. coli and instruct it to make a protein with the exact same chain of amino acids as in human insulin. So it's just like human insulin, but it comes from a bacteria instead of a human being."

"That's awesome," says Kevin. "Real Star Trek stuff." Kevin looks fine, and at breakfast I smelled no ketones on his breath.

Sometimes I wonder if this information is more than these folks need, but the more they know, the more comfortable about diabetes they will be, the more in control. There should be as few mysteries as possible.

Little Lucy is playing quietly with her Barbie Doll, but Emily is actually listening to me. So, is Inky, her black rabbit.

Pat asks another question. "Who besides Tate knows the brand of their insulin bottle?"

"Novo-Nordisk!"

"Lilly!" All the kids start shouting answers.

"Good," Pat says. "And you should know what brand you use and not mix them together or switch from one brand to another. In an emergency, it would be okay to mix brands, but in general it's a good idea to stick with the same brand and the same type, unless your doctor feels a change would help your control."

Pat goes on and explains about the expiration date on the bottle. We have certainly seen problems with expired insulin. It's important for the parents and kids to check this date. She teaches them our trick of putting clear tape over the expiration date, so that it cannot be rubbed off with time and use. Pat recommends always checking the expiration date when you buy it. "Make sure it won't expire before you are through with it."

"Pat, how long are insulin bottles good for once you start to use them, until the expiration date?" asks Darryl.

"No, the expiration date may be for two years but that is for unopened bottles. How long they last after being opened presents a problem to the pediatric population. The adults tend to use larger doses and empty a bottle more quickly. With little ones, like Emily who takes only a few units of regular insulin a day, that bottle would last a long time. Becky, how many units of insulin are there in one bottle of insulin?" As Becky thinks about this question, Pat motions to Eddy to leave the room. He must get ready for the next activity.

Becky looks at her bottle and frowns, "You mean total units?"

"Yes."

"There would be . . . 10 times 100, or 1,000 units."

"Right. So if you only use three units of regular insulin a day about how many days would a bottle last?"

"I know," says Kevin. "About a year or 333 days.

"Right, and that would mean twice as many sticks into the bottle if you were giving two shots a day. The drug companies have not made these bottle tops to be punctured 600 times. There would be a much greater risk of contamination from the multiple syringe pokes. Some companies recommend using the bottles for no more than a month. I think three or four months should be a maximum. And any time you see clouding in the regular clear insulin or clumps in the intermediate insulin, you should get a new bottle.

"Don't forget that insulin is temperature sensitive. It cannot be frozen, or it will lose its potency. Severe heat, like leaving it in the car in the summer, will also inactivate it."

"Does it need to be kept in the refrigerator?" Lydia asks. "That's what Kevin's nurse told me."

"The drug companies make different recommendations. If you keep extra bottles for future use, it's best to store them in the fridge. Or if it's very hot in your house in the summer, all bottles should be refrigerated. But you can leave it safely at room temperature, although that might shorten its duration of effectiveness. The problem is that cold insulin stings more than room temperature insulin. If you do keep it in the fridge, you can roll the filled syringe in your hands for a while, like this, to warm the insulin slightly. Pat demonstrates. "Any other questions?" she asks.

Heather gives Pat the high sign from the doorway. Pat continues. "Now, we're going to talk about injection sites, and, Eddy, our one and only Mr. Hulk, our Rocky, our Superman, will assist us."

Eddy comes through the door wearing a huge smile on his face and his fluorescent green and pink Speedo swimsuit on his body, which is well-tanned. The two little girls giggle, pointing to his hairy chest. Eddy jokes around, assuming a few body builder poses. Pat holds up two tubes of colored icing. "Who would like to show us where you can give your insulin injections?"

"Can I, can I?" asks Abigail.

"Sure, come on up. Mark a big X where you would give a shot." Abigail draws a large X with red icing on Eddy's thigh. Kyle marks the top of Eddy's upper arm (the deltoid area). Pat takes the opportunity to instruct. "Eddy has a lot of muscle in this area and it would probably not be the best spot to inject if you're looking for fat. It would be better to draw the X back here further." She draws a big gooey green mark on the back of his upper arm.

Other kids volunteer, putting gooey green and red X's on his abdomen, both sides of the belly button, and on the outer sides of his thigh. Little Lucy puts a big mark on Eddy's calf. Everyone chuckles. Everyone but Little Lucy knows that's muscle. Then, a few of the kids start to giggle and whisper. Pat and I know exactly what's going on.

Pat calls on Jeff, who says he can draw an arrow to the spot. Jeff tells Eddy to turn around, and then draws a big arrow on Eddy's back pointing downward toward his butt. Many parents prefer the buttocks, a relatively large area of fat, as an injection site for infants and children. It's a little hard for the older children to reach when they're giving their own shots, and sometimes its use is a source of embarrassment.

Having made an excellent model, Eddy, decorated with gooey icing, exits to the shower. Pat talks about the need to rotate injection sites. Always injecting into the same spot causes large lumps to develop, and the insulin is not well absorbed from these lumps.

"We call this *lipohypertrophy,* and it's important to keep a lookout for this." Again she emphasizes the importance of using different locations. "The reason some kids like it given in the same spot all the time is because it doesn't hurt after awhile. That's because the nerves have been damaged with repeated injections and local fat and insulin buildup."

"Kevin has lumps in his belly," says Lydia. Her son glares at her, and is not about to show the group his lumps.

I gently pull Jeff toward me. "If you run your finger over the leg or arm and meet a spot of resistance, this may suggest the beginning of lipohypertrophy." I demonstrate this on Jeff's bare thigh, but find no lipohypertrophy. He smiles, as does his mother.

Pat continues. "Injection site preferences seems to be very personal. How many of you kids like the belly best?" Ginny, Kevin, and Peter raise their hands. "How many like the leg best?" A few more raise their hands. And the rest prefer the arm or the buttocks. I comment, "I try to always ask which site is preferred and then check that spot. From my experience, if kids say they sometimes use their arms, it means almost never, or if they say they usually use their belly, it means always." A few parents and kids chuckle.

"Are there any questions about the things we've covered so far?"

Marjorie asks, "Does it really matter which site you use as long as you don't go into the exact same spot over and over?"

Pat answers. "Recommendations have varied on that. At first

some experts said you should rotate from arm to leg to belly. Then others said that blood glucoses are more consistent if you use the same area, but just not the exact same location. It's been shown that absorption from the abdomen is quicker than from the arm and from the leg and buttocks. But some feel this faster absorption is not clinically significant. Dr. MacCracken and I recommend that you use one location, say either thigh, for the morning and another location, say either arm, for the evening. This way you are consistent, but rotating, too.

I add, "Exercising an extremity will increase the insulin absorption. So if you're going to bike or run, the abdomen might be a better location than the leg. And another thing to remember is that increasing the temperature of the area of injection will increase the absorption. The insulin will have a quicker and stronger effect."

Mark comments, "I remember you told us about the teenager who had reactions after supper only on the nights that he used his hot tub."

Lisa, his wife, adds, "And the mother who said her baby was having reactions after breakfast. She figured out it happened on those days when she bathed her baby after breakfast."

"That's true. Those were practical situations that had to be worked out. Any other questions?"

"Are you going to talk about insulin action, the timing of different insulins?" asks Darryl.

"Let's do that after the break," I reply. Everyone heads out the door.

Kevin and Peter rush out to finish their pool game before any of the little kids move the balls. On the way I notice they each grab a cracker or two. After a shower, Eddy returns looking much less sticky. He knows what's next and doesn't want to miss it. Sam goes outside for his smoke, while the other adults have some more coffee.

After about 15 minutes everyone regroups and settles down. I draw some graphs on the board and proceed to discuss when different insulins work and for how long. I explain that the blood sugar tests done at certain times help us determine the appropriate insulin dose. The parents and, eventually, the kids need to learn to adjust the insulin dosage. I emphasize that we look for patterns and don't recommend making changes on just one value. I go over the duration of the different insulins. Most everyone has some idea about the difference between regular (short-acting) and NPH and Lente (intermediate-acting). Only a few parents are familiar with the long-acting insulins.

In the past ,these long-acting insulins have not been used too often in children, but times are changing and so are the durations of the newer human insulins. I try not to confuse them with too much information, but some of them read a lot about different insulin schedules. By the time I finish, I've done quite a bit of scribbling on the board. From their questions, I realize this subject isn't well understood. The 15 or 20 minutes we spend on this subject is very necessary. The parents, especially, learn a lot.

Pat announces that the next exercise may be difficult for some, but we strongly believe it's very worthwhile. The parents look at each other, anticipating our next words.

"It's a lot to ask these kids to take one, two, or three shots a day. You may be giving these injections, and many of you are eager for your child to give themselves their own shot. So, we feel that all of you should know how it feels to give yourself a shot," I say. A few parents are surprised. Their eyes show their fears and betray their secret thought. "You wouldn't make us do that, would you?" they question silently.

"Daddy, you can give yourself a shot," urges Susan.

"We've given each other injections in the hospital when Susan was first diagnosed," says Brent, relieved, as he looks at Marjorie.

"It's important for you to experience giving one to yourself," I add. "It's different than giving it to someone else."

"But I'm petrified of needles," whines Marjorie. Susan tells her mother it really isn't that bad. The kids enjoy this moment. Some even laugh at the fear of their parents. Think about it. Doesn't it seem only fair for parents to know what their children are experiencing. The real fact is that the fear of the needle is far worse than the stick itself. But it's not easy to convince someone of this at first. And the only way they'll believe that is to do it.

It's our policy that the parents must do this before leaving the hospital. Mark, Lisa, and Lucy have already done this exercise. But for the sake of the children and the other hesitant parents, all three are willing to do it again. Volunteering to go first, Mark grabs a new insulin needle, and after wiping a small area of fat near his waistline, he quickly inserts the needle. Just as quickly, he withdraws the needle and gives a great smile.

"Really, Marj, it doesn't hurt," he says kindly.

Lisa, sitting next to Mark, does the same thing. It takes her a bit longer to jab the needle into her thigh, but she does it and restates that it's hardly anything.

Now, it's Brent's turn. Susan stands by and encourages her father. "Daddy, you do me all the time. It really isn't that bad. Just pinch up the skin and go in."

He hesitates, "It's true. This is much harder." Brent wipes his thigh and waves his hand to dry the alcohol. "I had no problem injecting into the orange (an old hospital teaching technique) or Marjorie or Susan, but self inflicting pain is harder."

"Honest," I say, "you will be amazed just how painless it is." The parents or anybody who has never tried this have greatly inflated ideas of how painful it is, especially if your child has yelled and screamed when you do it. That yelling and screaming is usually from fear that later will be discovered to be unfounded, but the carrying on may continue for secondary gain. The old large needles of long ago simply aren't used for this anymore. The new needles are tiny and very sharp. But to the non-diabetics, the needle injection is thought to be about the worst part of the whole disease. From my experience, those with diabetes find the diet restrictions or the nuisance of finger pricking worse. And from this little exercise you can see that the fear is quite real for those who have never done it.

"Dad, really it won't hurt." Susan coaxes.

"Okay, Baby, if you say so," and he jabs it into his thigh. The expression on his face is one of relief and disbelief. "Did it really go in? I hardly felt it, really."

"See, I told you," Susan says proudly. Now it's her mother's turn. "Mom, Dad did it. You can, too."

"Yes, but Dad isn't afraid of them like I am." Marjorie looks at Brent for reassurance.

"Really, it's okay."

She takes a new needle from Pat, who is standing right by her side. She lifts her blouse and wipes a small area of her abdomen. She slowly waves her hand to dry off the alcohol. Marjorie looks determined, but very pale. As she pinches her skin, she takes a deep breath. Trying to prepare herself, she holds the needle close to her skin. Everyone waits. "God, this is hard," she says, hesitating. "How long do I have?" she chuckles, nervously.

"Oh, we'll wait here all day if we must," replies Pat, who puts her hand on Marjorie's shoulder and gently whispers, "Honest, it just isn't that bad."

"Boy, am I a chicken. Sorry, Suz, I must be embarrassing you."

"It's okay, Mom. You can do it."

Marjorie takes another deep breath and darts the needle into her skin. She leaves it in, and looks up. Her mouth is wide open, and her eyes reveal her utter surprise. "That was nothing. What was I so worried about?" This is the classic response, but, boy, it takes a lot of coaxing to get them to do the initial jab. It's definitely easier to try it on someone else. But everyone who deals with folks with diabetes should experience that first fearful jab. If parents with little children injected themselves first, then when they stick their child, they won't feel as guilty. They'll know it doesn't hurt that much.

With Jeff and Kyle watching, Lucy gives herself a shot like an old pro, but her fingers look stiff. I'm sure her arthritis is a lot more painful than this little needle prick. The two boys beam with pride. "Can I do it?" asks Kyle.

Pat says, "Sure, and hands Kyle a needle." Pat helps him pick a spot on his thigh and shows him how to pinch. Obviously, he has watched his mother do this to Jeff many times. He goes right in with no problem. Everyone applauds. Jeff is impressed.

Next in line is Lydia. She doesn't look too pleased with this project. "Dr. MacCracken, I can't believe you're going to make me do this. The nurses wanted me to do it when Kevin first got diabetes, but I hate needles and I refused. It looks like I got no choice now."

"That's right," I reply. "Kevin, tell your mother it won't hurt."

"Mom, it's gonna kill," he says with a big smile. Cindy watches her mother. Lydia slowly slides the needle into her abdominal fat. She doesn't appear to feel a thing.

"You're right, Brent, it wasn't too bad."

"Cindy, would you like to try?" Pat asks.

"Cindy don't like needles, neither," her mother states.

"Yeah, I'll do it," Cindy says, "but, can I do my arm?"

"Sure." Pat helps Cindy take a pinch of the back of her arm. Then Cindy pokes it in and out quickly. She's pleased. Her mother is surprised.

Pearl takes no time to go in and out and seems pleased to find out it isn't too painful. Of course, no one is injecting anything into the fat, and it may be slightly more painful with insulin in the syringe. But, still, the anticipation of pain is the major obstacle.

Becky has been observing everyone giving themselves shots. Is she enjoying this or is this little exercise destroying some of her sympathy getting material. Only her parents are left. Darryl holds the syringe and tells us about allergy shots his mother had to give him. He also remembers the large immunization guns they used in the Army. He's stalling but may be using this as a mechanism to prepare himself.

He too goes for the abdomen. We recommend a quick jab, but he places the needle on the skin and ever so slowly twists it in. We cringe, but he claims it's the way his mother did it. He's in and out. No wincing. Becky stands nearby, defeated. Nancy performs the operation with little effort. But I think she's amazed at how insignificant the needle stick is. I bet she felt her only child was going through hell twice a day with those injections. Becky won't be able to use this anymore.

Marjorie is still talking to Mark and Lisa about how scared she is of needles. Darryl asks Pat about the Inject-Ease, and Jeff demonstrates it to everyone. He does a good job. This kid is so mature for seven years. It's no wonder Steve and Lucy are so proud of their two boys. They bubble with enthusiasm and, luckily, it overflows onto the whole camp.

"Are there any questions?" Pat asks.

Kevin asks, "Pat, sometimes the insulin comes back out after I inject it. How come?"

"You have to take the pinch, insert the needle, release the pressure of the pinch, inject steadily, and then leave the needle in for a few second before pulling it out. If you continue to hold the pinch after you remove the needle, you can force some of the insulin out the tiny hole," she replies.

"And should you push the insulin in slow or fast, or doesn't it make any difference?" Brent asks.

Pat adds, "Again, it's personal preference. Some like it slow and others like it fast. It may depend on how large the dose is whether fast is painful or not. Any other questions?"

This morning has gone quickly. Lots of material has been covered. Another milestone, self-injection, has been accomplished. Step by step we are working to the home stretch. It's a beautiful sunny day, and I go sit on the porch steps to catch some rays and prepare mentally for this afternoon's individual family sessions.

From Science to Feelings

As Heather and I walk to lunch, we quietly start chanting our Indian song. This just may be a hit, or the audience may think we've flipped out. Certainly, anyone from the outside would. I suppose that's why we don't invite guests to the talent show. They wouldn't understand many of the in jokes, and their presence would probably inhibit a few campers who just might perform among their newly made friends.

At lunch Brent passes around some photos he had developed yesterday. He's captured some great moments; Pat, Heather, Tim, and Mark emerging after wrestling in the stream, Susan skating along on the mud in her flashy purple outfit, and Mark and Darryl trying to rescue Abigail's stuck shoe while keeping themselves out of the muck. They're priceless. Two snapshots stand out, one with Emily and Inky napping in Sam's lap. Sam's red hair is highlighted with the sun's rays. This would be a magnificent enlargement. The other captures Becky, Cindy, and Ginny, silhouetted against the pink and orange sky. It's lovely.

"Those are great, Brent. Can we get some copies? They'd be great in our album."

"Sure, I'll send you them."

Pat begins the announcements. "Dr. MacCracken, Heather, and I will be seeing families individually this afternoon. You rotate according to the schedule posted on the bulletin board. When your family is not scheduled to see one of us, you're free to participate in several other activities. Ginny will be located near the ping-pong table with materials to make our camp banner. We hope you'll all create something symbolizing your family, and then she'll attach it to the banner. I'm sure Ginny will help you with ideas, if you need some. The second activity is related to this evening. We'll be celebrating Pearl's birthday at a grand costume party."

"How old will you be, Pearl?" asks Kyle.

"Kyle, ladies don't tell their ages," says his mom.

Sam leans over and whispers in Kyle's ear. "Oh," Kyle says. Fifty's old to him, I bet.

Pat continues. "For costumes you'll find the makings in the attic in the big green chest. There are all sorts of get-ups including necessary accessories. Take turns going up there. Keep your costumes a secret. We'll ring the bell for you to go to your rooms to dress up around 5 or so and then ring it again for everyone to gather downstairs for our costume parade."

The announcements continue. "I've noticed a few more names on the talent sheet sign-up, but we need more. The more, the merrier. Kids, ask Ginny and Eddy for some ideas, and parents, let your inhibitions go. Let the performer come out in you. Don't be shy."

"What time will these afternoon meetings start?" Darryl asks.

"We'll begin at 1:30, so we can finish by about 4:30," Pat replies.

"The schedule says we have a guest speaker tonight," says Marjorie.

"Right, tonight after supper we'll have an eye doctor and his assistant tell us about the latest in prevention and treatment of diabetic eye problems. Dr. Takash from Waterville usually brings a movie and slides, and Paul, his assistant, works with the kids and teaches them about eyes. They arrive after dinner. But don't worry.

They know Thursday night is Costume Party Night and come prepared to see rather strange individuals walking around.

"If there are no other questions, Heather, Dr. MacCracken, and I will adjourn to our quarters until 1:30 to practice for our no-talent, talent show."

"What you gonna do?" Tate asks.

"Oh, that's a secret. What are you going to do?" Heather replies.

"Oh, that's a secret," laughs Tate, with that toothless grin.

Back at our cabin Pat says, "Once again, I hate to say this, but we've got a lot of work to do." About this time every year Pat starts to get worried. It's Thursday afternoon, and the week is rapidly going by. To draw everything together and have a successful conclusion does take a concentrated effort. Heather and I offer our help.

"What's the biggest thing we need to work on?"

"Well, by now, I usually have the awards pretty well worked out, but I haven't even started on them."

"Don't worry. We'll help you with that. This year will be easier than others."

"I don't know."

"Pat, you do a great job every year, this won't be any different." I really mean that. Pat has a special, sensitive touch when talking about people. Her caring always comes through. I suppose that's what draws me to her and keeps me wanting to do this crazy camp thing. Pat and I just click. Oh, we've had our times. I remember once when she was upset with me for something. I was oblivious to what I had done but keenly aware that she was not her usual self. But I never let anything like that last very long.

Once my college roommate told me I'm a tough friend to have because I'm so frank and open. Too true, I guess. I just say it like it is and don't even know how to throw the bull. Well, I went up to Pat and asked her what was wrong, and said I was sorry if I had done something to upset her. We talked it out, and that was that. An even closer bond was formed. In recent years, maybe because we work more closely together at the hospital, we've stayed in sync even better.

"I'll jot down a few suggestions this afternoon," I say.

"Me too," says Heather. "How about I be in charge of our costumes for the Indian chant. There must be something good in the attic, an old blanket or something."

"I've got these orange and yellow paper flames that we cut out for the campfire," Pat comments. "With a few snips they'd make great feathers for a headdress."

"Sounds good. I'll get some beads and wear my old Quoddy moccasins."

"Did you bring the clown outfits for tonight, Pat?" I ask. She nods. Pat's husband dresses as a clown with the Shriners. We've borrowed his outfits for the past few years, and the red sponge noses top off the costumes.

We practice our recorder songs, sing the Camp Kee-to-Kin song, and finish with the Indian Chant. Our rehearsal ends in laughing fits. The effort we put into these silly acts is worthwhile. It's our own version of psychotherapy. The last 24 hours haven't been too tough, but this afternoon will demand some insight and tact. Am I up to that?

It's 1:30 and no *Bangor Daily News* journalist yet. Quiet hour would have been a good time for an interview with some families. But newspaper people have their own time schedule. Heading over to the lodge, we notice two kites flying high. Peter and his dad work diligently keeping these aerials aloft. Mark's purple kite begins a nose dive.

"Run, Dad, run!" yells Peter, who gently tugs on his string and nurtures his kite in the winds. For a moment Mark's kite climbs, as he runs down the hill. But a final gust reverses the kite's direction, and it plummets into the grassy field. Peter's orange and yellow bulls eye kite now is a mere dot in the sky. Soon both start reeling in the strings, Peter's from above and Mark's along the ground.

Tate rides his bike round and round the porch. The little girls squeal in the wheelbarrow as Kevin, burning off some lunch calories, takes a tight corner on the porch. Too bad we can't write wheelbarrow rides into his daily routine at home. In the distance I hear singing and catch the final phrase, ". . . 'til you find your dream." Ginny informs me that Nancy and Cindy are practicing for the talent show, and Becky is secretly working on a clarinet piece.

The afternoon family sessions begin. Half an hour session each. For Pat, Heather, and me, it'll be three solid hours of teaching and answering questions. Half way through, we'll grab some juice. My meeting place is the gazebo. Away from the noises of the lodge, I can concentrate, and the children are less distracted. Sometimes it's only the parents I really need to talk with. I have Emily, Sam, and Pearl first, followed by Darryl, Nancy, and Becky, and then Peter and his family. Then juice. Then Kevin's family, Susan's, and finally, Jeff's.

Half an hour will not be enough for some of these families, but it's a start. All but Becky and Susan will be able to visit us on a regular basis at our clinic where we'll continue the education. Heather goes over their meal plans, taking individual likes and dislikes into account, as well as activity levels. She's skilled at suggesting meal plans that fit the child and the lifestyle of the family. Some families always eat at five, while others are more erratic. Some mothers love to cook, while others prefer fast food stops more often. Well-trained, up-to-date, tuned-in dietitians can make a difference. We're lucky to have Heather.

Sam helps me carry three folding chairs down to the gazebo. Emily runs ahead. Pearl walks behind. I notice Inky is coming to this meeting too.

"It is lovely out here," says Pearl. She looks out to sea. "Aroostook County is beautiful in its own way, but it sure doesn't have these saltwater views."

"I like the sea shells," Emily adds. She isn't whispering anymore. I remember my initial concern about her always whispering. I can't recall when that stopped here.

"It's a special place," I add, "and I'm glad you stayed to enjoy it." I take a look at Emily's blood glucose chart. Her levels have been fairly consistent, running a little high in the afternoon, but usually down by bedtime. Her dosage for her weight and duration of diabetes seems appropriate. Pearl has some questions regarding specific snacks, and I advice her to hold those questions for Heather. Sam wants to know about school and what they should watch for. Emily will be starting afternoon kindergarten in the fall.

"When she starts kindergarten, you want to be sure she has a good lunch and mid-afternoon snack. It's very important to prevent low sugars. The teachers tend to worry a lot at first and may or may not have had any first-hand experience with diabetes in their classroom. We have a handout you can give to the teacher, who should keep some glucose tablets in her or his desk. If this is the first group exposure Emily has had, she may catch a few more colds than she has while being just with you. She'll probably handle them just fine, but you should know what to do if she gets sick, doesn't want to eat, or has some vomiting."

Pearl says, "I remember her first ear infection. She was only two and didn't have diabetes yet. Her fever went so high. But antibiotics sure helped with that. I think she's only had two others, and they weren't so bad."

"She's been healthy for the last few years. I sure hope this school thing doesn't mess her up."

"Sam, most kids do fine, but a few more colds are likely. You'll just have to check for ketones and watch her sugars more closely if she gets sick. And like the work sheet says, if her sugars run high and she has ketones, she'll need some extra insulin. The first time through it, you should give your doctor a call to help you make your adjustments."

"Can we call you or Pat?" Sam asks.

"Sure, we'd be delighted to help you. And by the way, she may bring her colds home to you, too. So you, Pearl, and Ollie need to watch yourselves, too."

They have a few more questions about Emily, and then we focus on Sam's diabetes. Emily has been quietly playing with Inky and listens to our discussion of her father's diabetes.

"How do you think the two shots are working?" I ask. "It's only been a day, so perhaps you've noticed no difference yet."

"Well, yesterday afternoon was much better. And this morning my blood sugar was almost normal, and for years I know I've been high through the night. I wasn't checking, but I was getting up to pee a couple times a night. I slept straight through last night. It was great."

"Good. By Saturday morning we should have enough information to fine tune the dosage. And you'll have to adjust some when you get back and start working. I'm sure life here is a bit less rugged than your carpentry work."

"Yeah, banging in nails all day can burn calories." His tone of voice indicates a bit of sarcasm and frustration.

His mother comments, "Sam, honey, you know Ollie's willing to let you have more responsibility in the business as soon as you feel ready."

"I know, Mom. Nail pounding's all I was about up to doing. But I think I might be ready to help him in other ways."

"He'll be happy to hear that, Sam." They give each other that special mother-son look. Emily hasn't missed any of this. Maybe she and her dad will have more fun together now. She climbs up onto his lap and gets a hug.

"Sam, you should see an ophthalmologist. It is important for you to have your eyes checked at least yearly. Tonight, you'll hear more about that, but I would certainly recommend an appointment some time this summer. It would be just a baseline exam but really important, especially because you've had diabetes about what, seven years, and your control hasn't been that great lately."

"You're right, Doc. I'll come to Bangor to see the eye doctor, if Emily can come visit you and Pat and Heather. She's grown to like you folks."

"We'd love it. Any other questions before you move on to your next session?"

Pearl adds, "Do you think I should try the Inject-Ease on Emily? Jeffrey makes it look pretty easy."

"Why don't you ask Pat to show you how it works and see if Emily likes it better. We have a few more days to try it."

"Should we try that, Em?" Pearl looks at her granddaughter, comfortably sitting in her father's lap. Emily nods. Sam stands, realizing the 30 minutes are up.

As these three walk up to the lodge, I see Nancy, Darryl, and Becky coming this way. Their first day here flashes before me. Becky, the spoiled teen, who attacked her mother at every chance. The pregnant pause in the introduction circle, as everyone noted Becky's anger, directed at her mother. . . her parent's desperation and yearning for some miracle . . . Darryl's avoidance of the situation by taking more sales trips or diving into a gruesome Stephen King novel. And then, on Tuesday, Tim's clinical judgment of Nancy's depression and Pat's revelation of Nancy's suspicion of extramarital affairs on these long sales trips. Gad, this family needs help.

"Hi," is about all I can think of at this moment.

I move off the folding chair and sit in the grass next to the gazebo. Becky sits on the step; her folks join me on the grass. I direct my attention to Becky, for we haven't had much conversation except in my car on the trip to Ellsworth.

"Have you been growing a lot taller in the past year?" What I really want to know is if she has begun puberty yet. Girls grow rapidly in the early stage of puberty, so it's a good indicator. She's 12, going on 13, so ought to be into puberty, but sometimes girls in poor diabetic control are late to start.

"Her feet are certainly growing," says Nancy. "Those dress shoes we bought you this spring don't even fit anymore, do they?"

"Well, they were almost too small when we bought them." Becky says in a rather bitter way. It's not going to be easy to break this habit.

"If you're growing taller, you're moving into puberty, and during puberty the need for insulin increases, probably due to other hormones your body's beginning to make, like sex hormones and growth hormone. It doesn't imply that your diabetes is getting worse or that you're eating more than you should. Did you bring down your camp chart and blood tests from recent weeks?"

Nancy hands me Becky's camp chart, and Becky has no other blood test results. The first few days only a few tests were charted, but since Wednesday morning they've been recorded. She tells me that to be perfectly honest the values from the past few months would be worthless for me to look at because she made them all up just to please her parents. She's quick to say that sometimes she does them but forgets to record them. I ask her in general what those values were. Mostly high. She can't really remember the last time she's had a low reading, and over the past year her values are a lot higher than before.

"So, do you think I need more insulin?" Becky asks.

"It could bring many of your 200 and 300 readings down into a more normal range. In fact, you'd probably feel better with a lower overall blood sugar. But because you've gotten used to the 200s and 300s, it might take a while to get accustomed to a normal level. I'm sure, eventually, you'll notice you'll have more energy and just plain feel better. Let's increase your overall dosage by 10 percent. That shouldn't cause you any problem and then on Saturday, we'll see what effect that has."

Darryl comments, "She's on a total of 40 units now. You're suggesting she go up 4 more units?"

"Yes, for the first change I would just increase each dosage by one unit. So in the morning, give 19 NPH and10 regular and in the evening instead of 8 N and 5 R, give 9 N and 6 R."

Nancy looks over at Becky, but says nothing. "I've got it, Mom, 19 and 10 and 9 and 6."

At this point, I want some time alone with Becky, so I ask her parents if they would leave and give us a few moments to ourselves. Becky looks surprised, but her parents, look relieved—especially Nancy. As they head back up the hill to the lodge, I try to formulate my words carefully. Somehow, I've got to get her to ease up on her parents. If I say the wrong thing, she'll just clam up and turn a deaf ear. We all know people who may hear, but not listen.

"Becky," she looks over at me, "have you started your period yet?" She sits back just a little. Her frown and body language indicate her confusion. Was she expecting something else, like a lecture? Is she relieved to think I probably just wanted to ask such a simple question, but not in front of her father?

"Not yet, but I know all about it. My mother's told me about periods, but I already knew about that stuff. My best friend at school started this spring. She gets out of gym class on her first day." Her tone of voice changes when she mentions her mother.

"Periods can affect your blood sugars. Women vary in their responses, but most need more insulin just before their periods. It may be a few years before your period gets regular, but you should at least be aware of the effects diabetes can have."

Becky looks out to sea, perhaps brooding over all the "effects diabetes can have." I may have just lost her. Perhaps being direct might work.

"Becky, I've noticed that you have a tough time with your mom. Has that only been since your diabetes?"

She says nothing and continues looking at the water. Maybe she figures that if she says nothing, I'll stop. I'm still. The cry of a seagull breaks the silence. From the side I notice tears running down her cheek. She doesn't wipe them, as they fall to her shirt. Maybe this is what she needs. On Tuesday her mother cried. Perhaps it has taken a few days longer to lower Becky's thick defensive shield.

Ginny's been telling me that Becky's changing. I rise from my grassy spot, and sit down on the step right next to her. She sniffs and wipes her cheeks with the back of her hand. What's on her mind? Shouldn't everyone have someone to talk with? To confide in? Is the world too busy to listen to the inner feelings and thoughts of a hurting child. At least here at camp we ought to make the time.

Cautiously, Becky replies, "Really, Dr. MacCracken, I did hear what Sam said on Tuesday . . . about it being even harder to be a parent of a diabetic than a diabetic. I never thought of it that way. I just figure my mother needs to tell me what to do like she always has, but I guess she's been hurting, too. She's worried about me and about . . . ." She stops, possibly pondering if the next thought is too dangerous or if it is just too private.

"About your dad?" I guess.

Her tear-streaked face turns, and her eyes meet mine. "Yeah, about Dad. He's gone so much more now than he used to be. I know my mother blames that on me and my diabetes. Dad just can't handle it. And I miss him when he's gone and take it out on my mother. I just don't think they love each other anymore." Becky bursts into tears. I put my arm around her, and she leans over to be hugged.

It's so classic, yet each time so poignant. The brat, the snippy child or the caustic, abrasive adult, is hurting deep inside, needing to be understood, craving to share, perhaps wanting to change.

"It's a very scary thought that your parents don't love each other anymore. And even scarier if you think you're the cause." She rocks in my arms. I whisper, "I know how you feel." My heart pounds, as my throat tightens. The scene blurs as my eyes well up with tears. We slowly rock together.

With a deep breath, I start again. "Becky, I'm positive your parents love you and pretty sure they love each other. They just told me they're planning a second honeymoon." She sits up.

"They did?" she asks, timidly.

"They realize they need some time together alone. Sometimes lives can get too busy and confusing, and parents spend very little fun time together. Yesterday afternoon while you were with us in Ellsworth, they were finding themselves again, and I think they like what they found. Diabetes throws a monkey wrench, sorry that's an old term."

"My grandmother used to use it. I understand."

"Well, I mean diabetes can really cause tension and disruption in a family. It takes a lot of work for a family without diabetes to keep things going OK, and when diabetes comes into the picture, everything just gets much more difficult. It won't be easy, but I have a feeling you and your parents can work it out, change the cycle that has developed among you. Your dad tries to bury himself in his work and avoid the diabetes. Your mom worries too much about your diabetes and about her husband's absence. And you miss your dad and feel angry about your diabetes, your father's leaving, and your mother's nagging. And your fighting drives your father further away."

"That sounds about right."

"Well, your father is learning that he can't run away from your diabetes or his fears of diabetes. This week he has learned more about diabetes, and I bet he feels more comfortable with the decisions that need to be made. He also realizes how hard it's been on your mother, and wants her to get out and back into singing."

"Did he tell you that?"

"Yes, in so many words. And your mother has decided that she's been too uptight. She needs to let go some, but that's hard for her, especially if you won't take care of yourself. She just wants you to be as healthy as possible."

"I know. Ginny and I have talked a lot. She takes good care of her diabetes and is determined not to let it stop her. I can't believe she did that Outward Bound thing. I'd be too scared. But she says if I learn to take care of my diabetes, I would be able to sleep out on an island, too.

"Yeah, she probably told you you could be President of the United States, if you wanted to."

"Yeah, she did. She's going to be a lawyer, you know, and who knows maybe she'll run for President."

"She'd probably win, too," I reply. Becky finally smiles. "You've probably heard this before, but it really does have a lot to do with your attitude."

"Yeah, and Ginny sure has a positive one, that's for sure."

"So, your father and mother are trying out new attitudes and . . ."

"And maybe I should try a new one, too." She looks up for my comment.

"A great idea, and I have a feeling it may just feel better." I give her a squeeze, and she returns the hug. "Why don't you go find your parents and make a special family logo for the banner."

"I'll see if I can find them. See you later."

She walks quickly up the hill, as the next family starts down to see me. God, I hope that the cycle can be broken. It's hard enough to handle the stress of chronic disease. Throw the teenage years into the pot, where the battle for independence brews, and the stew may become just too thick. It's a delicate balance of so many things. The first three in diabetes are food, insulin, and exercise, but in adolescence there's also peer pressure, family interactions, puberty, school pressures, and those sex hormones. A tough, tough balancing act.

Mark and Lisa walk down the field. Peter and Abigail race towards me. Abigail hops on the platform, as her brother jumps on my back. We wrestle in the grass until his parents arrive.

"Hey, Pete, be careful of Dr. MacCracken," his mother gently reprimands.

"She's tough, Mom. Don't worry about her." We both brush off the straw. I tell Lisa that I've had a lot of experience with wrestling with my own kids.

I've enjoyed this family since I first met them six months ago in Bangor. They're a great addition to camp this year, and I tell them so. Mark and Lisa are pleased they came because Peter is having the opportunity to meet other kids with diabetes, and they are learning about some of the pitfalls they hope to avoid with diabetes in the family.

Though her little sister, Lucy, remains in the lodge playing, Abigail insists she accompany her parents and Peter to the meeting. As I go over Peter's glucose chart and the old records from home, Abigail listens intently. She really does want to be able to help with and learn even more about diabetes. I jot down on my mental list for awards night—Abigail, honorary nursing degree.

We talk about increasing Peter's insulin dosage. His blood sugars are slightly higher than they were two to three weeks ago. His current insulin dosage is still quite low. After pointing this out, we all decide that a little increase might be appropriate. Peter may always have a fairly low insulin requirement because he is so active.

In our clinics we definitely see the difference between the kids who are into lots of sports, maybe on a track team or swim team, and those who get no regular exercise. Besides having a healthier and happier outlook, they also seem to require less insulin. We encourage team sports as the kids get older and some regular exercise for the younger kids, like riding bikes or playing a game of backyard soccer. I recommend to all my patients, not just kids with diabetes, that less TV, less Nintendo, is always better.

Mark and Lisa ask specific questions and want me to check Peter's injection sites. He admits he doesn't like to use his legs at all. But he seems to be doing a good job rotating on his abdomen, and I don't see any significant lumps. His legs are solid muscle and injections can be more painful if there isn't enough fat to inject into.

Abigail wants to know what happens to all the syringes that the people with diabetes use. Now that's a great question from an eight year old and a dilemma for all of the adults. In the old days when the glass syringes and big metal needles were sterilized and used again and again, this question of disposal didn't come up. But just like so many things these days (plastic diapers, milk cartons, styrofoam coffee cups, etc.) insulin syringes with the built-in needles are discarded. Initially, when these plastic syringes first came out, people just threw them in the trash or in the toilet. But our society has had to face the issues of druggies reusing the syringes, trash men getting poked by the needle, a generalized fear of AIDS with blood contaminated needles, and the overwhelming question of disposal of waste.

Briefly, I give her our recommendation of collecting them in a plastic bottle (say a detergent bottle). There's even debate about whether you should break off the needle. Some feel there's a greater chance of sticking yourself. One answer for a collecting system may be inappropriate for all circumstances. But, obviously, we all want to avoid the medical waste from floating up on our beaches. Mark tells me that Abigail and Peter spend a lot of time cleaning up the beaches on Bar Harbor, and they are both acutely aware of the problems of trash.

Peter asks about the new, fluorescent orange blood glucose meters he has seen advertised in the magazines. He thinks they look awesome. We talk a little about the various meters, and I ask them to also talk to Pat about the new ones on the market. It's hard to keep up with the new turnover in meters. Companies continue to improve on their product. They get smaller, faster, easier to use, and, hopefully, cheaper and more accurate.

Overall, Peter's really doing very well, and he has an extremely supportive family. Both kids start pulling on grass shoots to chew on. We decide it's time for a juice break, and we stroll back up the field.

There's hustle and bustle in the lodge. Ginny, with Little Lucy's assistance, has been cutting out the banner. Heather's still talking with Kevin, Lydia, and Cindy, but Pat is taking her break, too. She comes over, and we talk briefly. She's just finished seeing Darryl, Nancy, and Becky. Of course, she wants to know what my conversation with Becky was all about, for Becky was fairly quiet in the session, but much more pleasant to her parents. I try to tell her the essentials. Time won't allow any more than that.

Lemonade hits the spot. I head back down to the gazebo to await the arrival of Kevin, his sister, and Mom. It's appropriate that Heather spend the most time with that family. They definitely need nutritional counseling.

The remaining three sessions go very well. I'm pretty forthright with Kevin about what he needs to change. We all openly talk about what happens when insulin is not taken. His mother seems relieved to know that these hospital admissions were not all her fault. Cindy's relieved this secret is out in the open. All agree that counseling with Tim would be a good idea.

Kevin doesn't want Lou at the counseling sessions. Lydia, with more grace and tact than I've previously noticed, agrees with Kevin. By no means are all the problems solved, but at least we have a start. And with this family that's all I can possibly hope for.

Brent and Marjorie come with Susan. Tate would rather bike ride. Susan's parents have a long list of questions written in Marjorie's notebook. They are disturbed by some of the discrepancies between my way of treating diabetes and their own doctor's. I go over my reasoning for disliking the sliding scale. I draw a graph to show my theory. I reexplain why I think looking for patterns is so important, instead of reacting to one abnormal blood glucose value.

Susan's blood sugars have been better since Wednesday, and she has had no further reactions. Marjorie says that this morning her daughter woke up and was ready to get up. That's a major change. I'm pleased with the progress that we're making. They seem to be, too. We have no problem filling the 30 minutes.

Finally, Lucy, Jeff, and Kyle join me. They've seen Pat and Heather and have very few questions left. That always happens with the last family. Part of it could also be that it is a little past 4, and everyone is about out of steam. Well, that can't exactly be the case, as I see Jeff and Kyle jump on and off the gazebo platform. We let them play.

Lucy and I talk about the week. She's eager to hear my opinion on her plan to reestablish the diabetes kids support group that fizzled out a few years ago in her area. I encourage her to begin again. Lucy asks me if it would be all right for Steve to come back on Friday night for the talent show. I make an exception and say yes. But he's not a real stranger.

We head back about ten minutes early. I'm hopeful the *Bangor Daily News* reporter has arrived, but there's no sign of her. Everyone seems very busy. As the other sessions wind up, the kids with diabetes start gathering around the table to check their sugars. Emily is right in there with the rest of them.

With tests completed, Pat rings the bell for everyone to go to their rooms to start getting their costumes ready. There they'll take their shots, too. We head back to our cabin to dress for the grand costume birthday party.

Bring in the Clowns

"Help me with my wig, would you? I can't quite get it on right."

"Turn it around," Pat says.

"Oh, that's my problem."

"MacCracken, you're too much," comments Heather. Perhaps the yellow wig along with the red and yellow striped pants and shirt are a bit showy.

"Yeah, well, you look sort of funny yourself with those big feet. Be careful not to trip." Her long black flipper-type shoes will be hard to walk in. Heather wears a blue wig with a red and white polka dot one-piece jumpsuit. It's huge. Pat uses a few safety pins to close up the unzipped back. For the past three years we have dressed up as clowns. It's easier than digging in the costume box, leaves more choices in the box for others, and presents a united staff—the three clowns.

Pat's umbrella and tiny hat top off her outfit. We all apply red lipstick to accentuate our mouths, and Heather gives herself a big black beauty spot on her left cheek. This year I decide to wear my sunglasses. When we are all ready, we don our noses, red foam balls with slits in them. They're light and stick on fairly well. The three of us head back down the driveway to the lodge to see the others' get-ups. Heather picks up her feet, thrusting them forward with each step. Are we crazy or what.

A car comes up slowly behind us. It can't be Dr. Takash. He isn't expected to arrive until after supper. Pat and Heather step to one side of the driveway and I, the other. I wave the car on and notice two women in the car. As the driver pulls up, I easily see the surprise on the driver's face. Rolling down her window, she speaks to a clown.

"I'm with the *Bangor Daily News,* and I'm looking for Dr. MacCracken," she says with a slight smile on her face. How would this clown know Dr. MacCracken?

"Well, looks like you made the right turn back there. This is Hersey Retreat, and believe it or not, I'm the infamous Dr. MacCracken on my way to a costume party." I take off my sunglasses and present her my white-gloved hand. As we shake, she laughs.

"This is not exactly what I expected to find."

Heather and Pat, my clownmates, introduce themselves to the passenger, the photographer. We tell them briefly about the costume party tonight and comment that we had expected them earlier in the day. The reporter apologizes. She had to cover a labor dispute at one of the mills, which took longer than she'd planned, and tomorrow her schedule is crazy, so it's this evening or not at all. As I invite them to view the parade and share dinner with us, my nose falls off. A nose such as this can work its way loose if you talk too much. Pat explains there will be time after supper and before our evening program to interview a few of the campers. Sounds great to them. They park and walk a little behind us to the lodge.

Eddy, clad in a long black robe with a white paper collar, immediately our camp priest, tells us the troops are getting restless in their rooms. "Then, Father Eddy," I say, "Ring the bell, so the others can come down."

The bell releases the hoards, and the costume parade assembles. We stand outside. First out the door are Jeff and Kyle, dressed as ladies. Kyle's blue dress, with white cuffs and a large white collar, hangs down to his feet, which are adorned with high heels so large he can barely walk. His woven, pink Easter bonnet has seen better years. And under his arm, he carries a wicker pocketbook. He and Jeff giggle, as they try to strut around. His brother has selected a red sun bonnet to match his stunning red and white tiered skirt, supported by a stiff petticoat. The centerpiece of Jeff's outfit, however, is the lacy blouse and its support beneath— probably socks stuffed into a bra. Both boys are howling while we enjoy their antics. Their mother, who has come out on the porch dressed in men's black dress trousers, leather shoes, and a hideous plaid sports coat with a flowered tie, laughs and laughs at her two little boys. At this point they are the true clowns.

Others follow, and everyone seems joyful in this celebration. Pearl, who is the guest of honor at this evening's birthday party, has elected to wear the full length white chiffon gown, which has definitely seen better days, but on Pearl it looks quite lovely. The first time I saw this gown was at our initial costume birthday party, which was in celebration of a young camper turning 16. I'll bet she'll never forget her sixteenth birthday, and I'm sure Pearl's fiftieth will be equally as memorable.

Emily and Little Lucy have both been staring at the three clowns. It's obvious they're not exactly sure who we are. The wigs and make-up, not to mention the baggy outfits, do conceal our identities from the younger kids. Heather bends over to talk to Emily, as she exams Heather's big feet. Pat turns on her battery operated bow tie, and it goes round and round.

Darryl, Nancy, and Becky come out together. Nancy wears a white painter's cap backwards and a plastic play stethoscope around her neck. She carries a Fisher-Price medical kit. A white lab coat, green surgical pants, and green shirt complete her outfit. A yellow hand-made name tag, Dr. Quacken, identifies her professional character.

Darryl, not to be outdone, has his name tag, Nurse Stinger—a coincidental likeness to Pat's last name of Stenger. The red turban, white pants, and pink cotton dress, which is a bit tight around Darryl's shoulders, are definite fashion setters. Both seem pleased with their creations. Becky, completing the mock staff, has a black wig and an gaudy orange hat with artificial grapes and bananas on the top. In each pocket of her gigantic brown sweater are cookbooks. And the nametag—Ms. Exchange, RD. These folks take the cake for originality.

Every year someone finds the old lady's bathing suit, and it's never a lady who wants to wear it. We've had boy counselors and even fathers put on this awful yellow, black, and white suit. This year Kevin claims it. He fills it out in the hips and a bit too much in the stomach, but relies on tissue, I think, for the chest expanders. I get a kick out of watching Cindy laugh at her brother as he tries to strut like a Miss America contestant. We all applaud and hoot.

It's just a fun time. Another release valve. One year a boy put on a brown garbage bag that covered all his clothing, creating a California Raisin. We get cowboys and clowns, ballerinas and bag ladies, doctors and Dolly Partons. The same assortment of clothing with different imaginative combinations.

We take family photos for our album, and Brent snaps several, too. The newspaper photographer snaps a shot of the whole group, and then we promenade to the dining hall.

Twisted streamers of red and white crepe paper decorate the dining room, providing a festive air. Red paper tablecloths cover our usual daily plaid oil cloth coverings. And a huge banner, stretching from one end of the room to another, says, "HAPPY BIRTHDAY, PEARL—WE LOVE YA!!" She's surprised. It's probably been a few years since she had such a celebration. Her son and granddaughter beam. They sit on either side of her, as the rest of the campers grab seats.

My head itches with this wig, but I suppose I can stand it. But eating with my foam nose on is too much. Heather and Pat remove their noses, too. We look silly enough with the big red smiles. Pat and I sit with the newspaper reporter and photographer, who appear overwhelmed with the merriment.

"You all seem to have fun here. But I guess that's what a camp is for. Do you have education, too.?"

Pat replies, "Oh, yes. We try to educate almost all the time. But it can be subtle at times." We continue to talk through dinner. The reporter is intrigued with the idea of family camp. I tell her I have always hoped that someone would visit at the very beginning of the week and then return at the closing and make their own conclusions about the effects of the week. She thinks that sounds like a great idea, but admits it may be more than a newspaper would do. Perhaps, a magazine feature story.

"Or perhaps, "20/20" or "Sixty Minutes," Pat suggests. She's been interested in doing a film on the camp, but we just haven't gotten around to it. We've experimented with our camcorder, but we'd need professionals to do the filming. Maybe someday.

"I'd love to interview a few of the families after dinner. Could you see if there are any volunteers?"

"Sure."

As the dinner dishes are being cleared, Pat stands and introduces our Bangor guests. She asks for volunteers to speak with them, and several parents and kids raise their hands. Then she says that the dessert will be served in a moment, but first it is time to sing "Happy Birthday" to Pearl and have her say a few words.

The rendition is, at best, united, barely harmonious, but genuine, to be sure. Abigail has been given the responsibility of presenting Pearl with a big card signed by everyone. She completes her mission as we finish the second verse. Everyone applauds and cheers. Pearl looks at Sam and Emily and then stands up.

"I really appreciate all you've done for my birthday. I wasn't looking forward to this one—50 seems pretty old to me." Emily giggles. "But you've all made it very special. I feel in this short time we've become extra-special friends, and that's the best way to spend a birthday. Thank you all very much." As she sits down, she gives Sam a hug. Everyone applauds again.

"Will you really have birthday cake?" asks the photographer. She must know something about diabetes.

Heather announces that for our birthday celebration Laurie has made angel food cake, and we'll top it off with fresh strawberries and whipped cream. A regular strawberry shortcake delight. All the kids clap. Thank goodness, for the nondairy, low-calorie topping. And the fresh strawberries are yummy.

The Eyes
of the Beholders

After the gala birthday party we walk back to our cabin to change out of our clown outfits. "That was a fun party," Pat comments. "Emily and Little Lucy got such a kick out of our costumes. Lisa said her daughter had never seen a real, live clown before."

"I thought she was going to cry when Heather's nose fell off. But actually she enjoyed helping put it back on," I add.

Heather quips, "You know, I could get used to this life. Do you suppose the hospital administrators would employ a nutrition clown?"

"Couldn't promise you that," Pat replies.

It feels good to remove the itchy wig. The lipstick comes off fairly well with cold cream, but we all still have a hint of large rosy lips as we head back to the lodge.

The newspaper reporter is talking to Brent and Marjorie. Tate and Susan stand by their parents. At supper the reporter told me she'd like to talk to a family from Maine and one from another state. Peter and his family wait in the wings for their turn.

"Dr. MacCracken, how about that game of ping-pong," says

Kevin, who has exchanged the lady's bathing suit for his torn jeans. He's been waiting to challenge me again.

"Sure, you're on, Kevin." As I enter the playroom, I see Jeff, Kyle, and Sam at the pool table. Ever since Sam carried their mother out of the Fort Knox caves, these two boys have been hanging around Sam, and Sam appears to enjoy their attention. Nancy, Becky, Cindy, and Lydia talk together near the popcorn machine. It's the first time I've seen all four of them together. Pat told me earlier that Nancy and Cindy are having fun together, practicing for the talent show.

Over by the fireplace Darryl chats with the counselors. Parents gravitate toward Ginny and Eddy for first-hand advice. Often parents hear that the teenage years are so tough with diabetes. Here we show them examples of some teenagers who are doing pretty well. Neither of them would say it's easy, but neither plan to let diabetes stop them from their life goals. I think back to the movie, "Focus on Feelings" and the reference about having the option to pick up the paddles (the tools to help control diabetes) and guide your boat versus just drifting, aimlessly. These two kids are planning to actively work for what they want. Diabetes will be no disability to them.

"Dr. MacCracken, serve 'em up."

"OK, Kevin. You ready?"

"Ready as I'll ever be," he says. I'm sure he won't realize I'm playing left-handed. After we finish two close games, Abigail comes running in and tells Pat that two men are walking down the driveway.

"Kevin, we'll have to stop now. Our guests are here. Shall we call it a tie?"

"Sure," he smiles.

Pat and I walk out to meet Dr. Takash and Paul, his assistant. We're old friends, for they have come as guest speakers for several years. Parents have enjoyed their presentation, and the kids are always intrigued at seeing the inside of an eye. Both men donate their evening to do this, and in return we give them, as a token, a special camp T-shirt for themselves or occasionally their children. But their greatest gratification is in knowing that a few more families with diabetes have learned to appreciate what can be done to prevent the complications of eye disease in the people with diabetes.

As we walk toward the front door, our other visitors tell us they must be on their way back to Bangor. The reporter says she'd love to stay for Dr. Takash's talk, but she must get back. She thanks us for our hospitality and the opportunity to share in the festivities.

"This will be an exciting story to write," she says.

"When do you think the article will appear in the paper?" Pat asks.

"Maybe Saturday or next Tuesday in the life-style section. I can't be too definite."

"Well, thanks for coming," Pat and I say, simultaneously.

"We'll be watching the papers, and remember that left turn at the stop sign," I add.

"Thanks."

"Bye, bye," yells Tate, who obviously enjoyed being interviewed and photographed.

Inside, Paul and Dr. Takash set up the slide and movie projectors. We use the big white shade as our screen. I introduce our guests to the campers. Dr. Takash suggests that the kids go with Paul, while the parents watch a movie and then some slides. There will be time for questions during and after the movies. Eddy and Ginny stay with the adults, and Pat and Heather assist Paul with the kids. Emily grabs Pat's hand, and they exit with all the rest of the kids.

In general at camp we don't talk about complications too much. We try to dispel fears and mistaken information, but we purposefully don't harp on problems. First of all, we just don't see complications in children. We'd be talking about things down the road. And secondly, there just are not good statistics out yet on complication rates in children who have had the advantage of blood glucose monitors.

The large study recently completed has given us some solid information regarding control and complications. Quite a lot of recent information on the structural damage to nerve cells and kidneys can be related to hyperglycemia (high blood sugar). We feel our aim is to encourage the families to strive for the best control they can get, without, of course, allowing the pendulum to swing too far and cause frequent hypoglycemia (low blood sugar). This is a lot for them to be concerned with.

Treatment of diabetic eye disease, particularly diabetic retinopathy and macular edema, has advanced so much in recent years. We think it is very encouraging and reassuring to discuss this with the parents. Some of them have heard others talk or have read about blindness in diabetes. Many of these parents are too scared to ask. They don't want to know or imagine that their child could become blind. And yet others haven't heard anything about diabetes affecting the eyes. Both of these need to hear the accurate truth from Dr. Takash.

Last year, I recall that one parent was very relieved in hearing the presentation, and yet another parent was horrified. This was the first he had heard of these potential problems. I think most parents have heard about this complication and are afraid.

As the movie ends and the slides begin, I look around the darkened room. The parents are quiet, staring at the screen and sitting forward to catch every word.

Dr. Takash begins, "As the movie described, in diabetic retinopathy, abnormalities develop in the blood vessels in the retina, the back inner lining of the eye. These tiny vessels, which nourish the retina, may start to leak. In the early stages this leakage of clear serum can cause tissue swelling within the macula, the area of central vision. This swelling, called 'macular edema', can cause blurring of the central vision. Usually, the serum is reabsorbed into the neighboring blood vessels, and the swelling lasts only a few days. But if the leakage is too fast, the edema (swelling) may last longer."

He moves on to the next slide. The reddish color of the enlarged retina on the screen casts a glow over the room. "The tiny blood vessels can also bleed. Vision is not usually affected because the hemorrhages (bleeds) tend to be small and rarely occur in the central area. The goal of treatment, as the movie said, is to save the central vision area, the macula. The laser has been found to be able to seal these leaking vessels to prevent further edema and bleeding."

The next slide shows a retina with small, white, circular dots on its surface. These are the laser spots, tiny little laser burns, aimed at the leaking vessels. This slide reminds me of the tour we give the children and their families through the laser treatment room at Eastern Maine Medical Center. Our local ophthalmologist performed a pretty fancy trick to show the kids what a laser could do. She pulled out a one dollar bill and attached it to the machine. As we watched with our protective goggles on, she fired the laser gun at George Washington. Of course, we heard nothing but saw a flash of light. The eye doctor then had us pass the dollar bill around and look closely at Washington's eye. Holding it to the light, we could see a pin point hole right through the President's pupil. What a shot! It showed the kids how small the burn is and how accurate you can be with the laser gun.

Dr. Takash continues. "We are now able to prevent much of the blindness that once was quite common in people with diabetes. The early diagnosis of retinopathy is most important. That is why we strongly suggest that your children have yearly ophthalmologic examinations, starting about five years after the diagnosis. Nothing may be visible for several years, but it is important to have a baseline and also to establish the habit of seeing an eye doctor yearly. In diabetes, prevention of progressive retinopathy is very important."

"Can a person with diabetes tell something is going on in their eyes?" Darryl asks.

"This bleeding and leakage is painless. A visual change is noticeable only if the central visual area is affected. And that can be a blurring, or even worse, total loss of vision in that eye," Dr. Takash replies.

"Kevin complains of blurry vision when his blood sugars are high. Is that retin . . . retino . . . ."

"Retinopathy," Dr. Takash assists Lydia. "No, probably not. There can be blurry vision when you have fluctuations in the blood glucose, and this can cause the lens to change shape."

"So, that's why Susan's eye doctor didn't want to give her a new prescription when she first came down with diabetes. He said we should wait a while until things settled down," Brent comments.

"That's correct," comments Dr. Takash.

The questions continue for some time. Our guest handles them well. Not just diabetes, but the whole field of eye disease seems to get covered. It's a free for all on an ophthalmologist— a rare opportunity for interchange.

The discussion concludes only when a few of the younger kids start coming in looking for their parents. I assume it must be snack time, when Little Lucy enters carrying her peanut butter covered graham crackers.

"Thank you very much," says Brent, and all the parents join in a round of applause. The parents pick up the hand-outs from the table, and most head out to find their kids.

Eddy talks with Dr. Takash, who has checked Eddy's eyes for several years. So far, there've been no problems. And I'll bet Eddy plans to keep it that way. The sad part of the story, which I have heard from Dr. Takash, is that so many folks with diabetes don't come for check-ups. They assume there's nothing wrong because they have no pain or visual problems. And then one day, all of a sudden, one of those abnormal blood vessels ruptures and bleeds into the inside of the eye, totally blocking the light that normally goes to the retina. Then, the person can't see and goes to the doctor. But by then much damage has been done.

There may be resorption of the blood over a long period of time, but when you have a big bleed like that, it means there are probably lots of damaged blood vessels just ready to rupture too. Extensive laser therapy may be able to save the central vision. But if only that person had gone for regular check-ups, it could have been prevented. Blindness from diabetes does not have to occur.

Paul comes over to put away the slide and movie projectors. He appears to have survived the children's session and tells us the large plastic eyeball was again a big hit. Everyone had the opportunity to take it apart and reassemble it. So they all learned the parts of the eye and where the lens goes. He used an old camera to show the similarities between the eye and a camera. Paul admits it got a bit too technical trying to explain how the film in the camera gets developed.

Heather comes in to join us. "Did he tell you what Abigail said?"

"No, not yet," says Paul. "Why don't you tell it."

Heather loves a good story. "Well, Paul was sitting in the rocking chair with a small chair next to him. He had each child sit down next to him, and then he looked into their eyes with an ophthalmoscope. He had examined several of the kids, and then it was Abigail's turn. She sat down beside him. Because she was sitting a bit far away, Paul placed his hand on her shoulder and leaned her forward to look into her eye. All of a sudden she said, 'Ouch, you're hurting me'. Paul explained gently that looking into your eyes shouldn't hurt. Abigail responded, `No, but you're rocking on my toe.' All the kids laughed, as Paul rocked off Abigail's toe. I suppose you'd have to have been there to get the real picture."

Paul adds, "She was so polite about my being on her toe, and all I could think of was her eyes. But besides that small incident, I think it went very well. There may be some budding eye doctors out there."

"Or photographers. They did like the camera," adds Heather.

"Paul, we'd better be going," Dr. Takash states.

"Well, thank you so much for coming again. I know the parents enjoyed hearing you and seeing the films. It's wonderful that they had so many questions."

"They were good questions, too."

"Would you like some juice before you go?"

"No thanks. We should be heading back."

I give them their well-deserved Camp Kee-to-Kin T-shirts and walk them out to Dr. Takash's old style green Chevy convertible. It's a beautifully warm, starry night for the drive back to Waterville.

Back in the lodge, the kids are recording their blood sugars on the charts. I quickly look them over to see if anyone needs a larger snack. Most of the results are pretty good. Peter is still a little high tonight, but we'll give the new insulin dosage a chance before increasing further. Mark and Lisa agree with that suggestion. Mark has his youngest daughter in his arms and heads up to bed. Peter, Abigail, and their mom follow. As I look around for Pat and Heather to head back to the cabin, Emily, carrying her stuffed rabbit, runs straight for me. She informs me that both have brushed their teeth and want a good-night kiss. I give Inky one on the top of his furry head, and Emily gets one on her cheek. I get a big hug. She runs off to Pearl, who is waiting at the staircase.

"Good night, Pearl," I add. "Sleep tight." Emily waves as she goes upstairs. Sam is just behind them and waves, too.

I don't see Pat. Heather comes toward the door and tells me that Pat and Eddy are having a conversation, which might take awhile. We decide to head back to the cabin to wait for Pat. We've lots to get done before bed tonight.

"This has been a great week for recipes," Heather says, as we walk along the driveway.

"Really?" I respond, not knowing exactly what she means.

"Yeah, Lisa and Lucy both like to cook, and it's been fun trying to help them adjust their casserole recipes to be better for Peter and Jeff. It's fun when mothers want to be inventive and experiment.

Remember Lil? She loves bringing us those special muffins in clinic. Diabetes just can't keep a good cook down, you know."

Heather and I switch on the lights and drop our things on the table. She sits down on the couch and automatically reaches for her knitting. The dog sweater is progressing slowly. But then, it's only June; cold wintry nights are far off. I find my reading glasses and look over the words to our songs. While waiting for Pat, we decide to memorize the words, and we also play a few rounds on our recorder. All the while, I'm thinking about Eddy. He's done so well here. I wonder if he's still upset about his little sister getting diabetes. I'm sure that's what Pat is talking to him about. Well, we'll find out soon.

"Remember the year we gave out the "You've Come a Long Way, Baby" Award? I think Becky could get that this year, but the Virginia Slims Advertisement isn't well known anymore, and they might not understand. Well, we'll just have to think of another phrase."

"Pearl will be easy. She's been a wonderful grandmother to all the kids."

"Yeah, and she's learned a lot about diabetes, too."

"So, what about the All Ears Grandmother Award?"

"Somehow, that doesn't sound right, think a bit harder."

Pat, who quietly walks in, hears our conversation. "How about Most Knowledgeable Grandmother Award?"

"Yeah, that's better. How about Most Knowledgeable and Supportive Grandmother Award."

"Great!"

"How far have you guys gotten?" Pat inquires.

"Well, we've memorized our words and practiced our recorder tunes, and we've just started talking about the awards."

"Well, let's go family by family. It's easier that way."

"You guys want a soda before we attack this delicate task?"

"Sure, and bring some crackers, too."

For the next hour and a half we talk about the families, about their progress and accomplishments. We laugh about the funny episodes of the week. Of course, it's impossible not to reminisce about the other years and the wonderful people we've gotten to know here. Where else can a millionaire and a blueberry packer laugh and cry, side by side? Or a Wall Street executive push a marshmallow across a floor with his nose?

After we essentially complete the list of awards (there are always a few changes after field day), we run through the songs. While choreographing our new song with Chief Somogyi and the Rebounds, we start to get punchy. The three of us erupt into uncontrollable laughter. Will we be able to be serious enough to perform our new act? We hope so, but if not, then the audience will just laugh along with us.

Twelve o'clock again. Time for bed.

Crawling into bed, I remember Pat's conversation with Eddy. As she comes out of the bathroom, I ask, "Is Eddy OK, Pat?"

"He's fine. He's had such a good time that he doesn't want it to end. He's really gotten attached to the kids, especially Tate and Peter and is concerned about what will happen to everyone, like Becky, Susan, and Cindy. Eddy's a great kid. He just needed to talk it out a little."

"Did he say anything about his sister?"

"He said that seeing these other younger kids with diabetes has actually made it easier for him to accept his sister's diabetes. Hearing Sam talk about Emily's diabetes made him understand some of his own feelings. He's going to be all right."

"That's good. We had hoped he'd get something out of returning to camp, and it sounds like he has."

"Yeah, he was a good choice—gets involved just like the rest of us." She clicks off the light. "Good night, Joan."

"Good night."

Back to the Future

As I stand under the warm spray of the shower, I think about the day ahead. Friday, our last full day of camp. Today will be packed full of activities. All our work will be essentially completed tonight. Tomorrow morning will just be breakfast and good-byes.

Today we'll try to answer any remaining questions. There will always be more we can do, but, in a way, this week should be just a new beginning, a new start for some families. If that is what we have provided here, then we've done our job. I'm still concerned about Kevin.

"Joan, save a little hot water for me," Pat insists.

"I'll be right out." Shutting off the water, I reach for my towel and dry off. I pop in my contact lenses. "Sorry, about that, I was deep in thought in the shower."

"Yeah, I know. We're certainly headed down the final stretch. I'll take a quick one and be right with you."

About this time, I start thinking of my family. It's been six days since I've seen them. Bob called once. He sounded tired. Luckily, both kids are having fun at soccer camp. Now that they're bigger, it's easier to leave them. But this week has always been tough because it's so all-consuming for me. My daughter used to come with me to camp; it was fun to have her here. But, after seven years she decided to do something else. While she was here, she learned so much about diabetes that we gave her the title of Junior Counselor. The last two years haven't been quite the same without her. Pat misses her a lot, too. Maybe next year she'll come again.

I make my bed and try to pack up my papers. Once again I haven't gotten to my filing of articles. I always plan on reading and getting other work done, but I never do.

Pat pokes her head around the doorway. "It's 7:15. Let's head over to the lodge. Here are the tests and the evaluation forms for the parents. You'll need them this morning."

It's cooler than yesterday, and the dew sparkles on the freshly mown grass. The hot muggy days of July have not yet arrived.

Sam sits on the porch railing having his morning cigarette. It takes all the restraint I can muster not to tell him about smoking and its detrimental effect on folks with diabetes. I just read that smokers have earlier problems with protein spillage in their urine, besides more vascular problems.

Someday, soon, I'll talk to him about it. But, trying to get him to drop that addictive habit would be too big an intrusion into his privacy now. I'm just so glad he stayed through the week..

"Doc, great morning. Can't beat this Maine sky," Sam says.

"My sentiments exactly," I reply. "I guess the predicted weather front must have blown through or gone south. I'll take a few more days just like yesterday."

"Me too." He exhales a cloud of smoke.

Jeff, now standing next to Sam, asks if we can do the water slide again. Pat promises this afternoon would be a good time. Jeff asks Sam if they can ride down the slide together. Neither Emily nor Sam tried the water slide on Tuesday, but now with his encouraging, new young friend Jeff, Sam agrees. A huge smile comes over Jeff's face.

Blood testing, breakfast, and announcements go well. As a group, we've all pretty much fallen into an easy routine. On the way back to the lodge after breakfast, Marjorie and Nancy agree that having the meals all prepared is quite the luxury. Jokingly, they quip that perhaps they'll stay for a few more weeks. Life is quite easy and relaxed here.

At 9 o'clock, the morning session begins. The parents and I go to the meeting room while Pat and Heather take the kids to the attic. There's a certain fascination with the attic with all its nooks and crannies.

We grab seats and form a small circle. I begin. "You've been asking me about the research that's going on in diabetes. There are several different areas of research. Many centers are exploring the causes of diabetes.

"In Pittsburgh they're looking into the geographical differences that occur in the incidence of diabetes. Perhaps that holds the key to explaining the cause—or a cause. We know there appear to be multiple factors in the equation of cause. Researchers continue to probe these areas.

"We want to know what role viruses play, or environmental toxins, or certain foods we eat. Why, for example, do babies who are not breast-fed get diabetes more often than breast fed babies? Why does diabetes tend to occur in seasonal peaks? Are certain foods bad for you? Why do the Scandinavian countries have so much more diabetes than the Japanese? Just what is the trigger that stimulates the pancreas to self-destruct?

"All these questions are being explored, but no answers are evident—yet. Molecular biology probably holds the key to these answers, and scientists are delving deeper and deeper into molecular science.

"More directly related to your families, though, is the research in the area of new treatments and prevention. I want you to know that I feel very strongly that the day will come, and in the not too distant future, when diabetes will be prevented. We will be able to screen individuals, and if they are identified as being at risk, protect them from developing the disease. So I think diabetes will be preventable in a large number of people.

"For those who already have diabetes, there will be some very sophisticated treatments. I think we'll have some sort of an insulin infusion pump that can be implanted and sense the body's need for insulin without the individual having to do finger sticks all the time.

"I don't think there will be an actual cure for diabetes. I mean, the pancreas of people with diabetes will probably never be repaired, but some form of artificial pancreas will be developed that will replace the damaged one."

"All of that is encouraging, but just how far away do you think we are from these things you've mentioned?" asks Mark.

"I can't possibly predict that, but so much progress has been made in the last decade that I think the next decade or two will be the crucial time. It will be in your children's lifetimes."

"Can you predict if someone is going to get diabetes?" Lydia wonders. I think she's learned a lot here. I've enjoyed educating Lydia this week. She's been an attentive student. The more you give these folks to work with, the better they can handle it.

"Lydia, researchers have shown that in most patients with diabetes it takes quite a while for the symptoms to show. In fact, about 90 per cent of your pancreas must be destroyed before increased urination and thirst occur. This destructive process appears to be going on for weeks, months, or even years before any symptoms arise. But this destruction is an *autoimmune* process. What I mean is that for some reason the pancreas is being attacked by certain immune cells in the person's own body. Thus, the word 'autoimmune'—an actual self-destruction."

"And they can measure the destruction as it is progressing?" asks Brent.

"They're getting more accurate at interpreting their findings of autoimmune products, referred to as antibodies. They also study the remaining function of the pancreas by measuring what is called 'first phase insulin release' during an intravenous glucose tolerance test. This test indicates whether the pancreas is losing its ability to perform correctly. In fact, a few researchers now believe they can predict how long it will be before the symptoms of diabetes occur by knowing these antibody levels and the results of the intravenous glucose tolerance test. Others don't think it's quite that easy."

"The Joslin Clinic is involved in this, isn't it?" asks Pearl. "My sister-in-law lives in Boston, and she wrote me about this research they're doing."

"Right, Pearl. The Joslin Clinic and nine other clinical centers are now involved in a national study called the Diabetes Prevention Trial. This study hopes to identify people before they come down with diabetes by screening them for elevated antibody levels."

"Will they test anyone?" Marjorie asks.

"To be eligible for the study you must be between the ages of 4 and 45 and have a relative with Type I diabetes, preferably in the immediate family, though they will do cousins, aunts, and uncles if they are under 20."

"What if they have antibodies," Nancy queries?

"Then further testing is done. If that's positive, then they have an opportunity to enter the study where they will be randomly assigned to the experimental or the control group. The experimental group takes very low doses of insulin and checks their blood every once in a while. I have some handouts with more details if you're interested. It's still just an experiment. No one knows if we can prevent the onset of diabetes with insulin, but it is the first big study. They want to screen about 60,000 people. Maybe you remember me saying that only 3 to 6 percent of immediate relatives will get diabetes. And many children who get diabetes don't have any relatives who have it."

The parents share their family stories. It's great to hear them all participate. I always wish research would be faster. We seem to wait so long for the next piece of the puzzle. But research must be carefully done by cautious scientists. However, I can still give these folks the brighter side of the diabetes picture.

"Have they tried other ways of giving insulin, besides shots?" Sam asks. He has changed this week. I hope we'll stay in touch. Emily has blossomed, and Pearl has gained so much more confidence.

"Sam, some people have tried to develop a coated pill that would not be digested by the stomach acids. I don't think much has come of that. Others have tried nasal sprays. There are hormones that can be given by nasal spray, but when you get a cold, you can imagine the erratic absorption. Recently, I read about seeing if insulin could be infused through the skin using an ultrasound device. Animal studies have been done, and I think they are starting human trials. We'll have to see."

"Aren't they working on transplanting pancreases?" inquires Darryl. "An old roommate of mine from Minnesota wrote to me about that on his Christmas card. Nancy and I thought it a rather strange Christmas message, but you know how friends are always giving suggestions." The group collectively chuckles. I guess friends are always trying to help.

"Minnesota has been the hot bed for pancreatic transplantations. Most of those have been done on patients who have already had kidney transplants because of renal failure from diabetes. They are already on immunosuppressive drugs to suppress rejection of the kidney transplant, so the risk of pancreatic transplant would not involve adding suppressive drugs. Does that make sense to you?" Most nod. I continue. "Most of these transplants are from cadavers, although recently there have been a few live-donor, partial pancreatic transplants. But the expense and risk does not really make that a practical therapy for all the folks with diabetes."

Marjorie comments, "I read somewhere, I think it was in the *New York Times,* about beta cell transplants."

"That's certainly being worked on. Researchers are trying to discover how to hide these transplanted cell so the body will not reject them as foreign. They've implanted donor beta cells into the liver and have enclosed them in a net to protect them. It may be a feasible therapy. Harvesting these beta cells is very time consuming, though. Techniques to use islet cells from animals are being investigated. My feeling is that soon some sophisticated, computerized, miniature pump that can be set to infuse insulin will be developed. This will be monitored by another sophisticated, sensitive, miniature sensor. Or they'll use beta cells and hide them in protective filaments. Really, if we can put a man on the moon and then bring him back to within a few miles of a ship in the middle of the Pacific Ocean, we should be able to develop the mini-machine I'm talking about."

"I agree!" proclaims Lucy.

Everyone starts to talk to the person next to them. It does seem that scientists with modern technologies ought to be able to do this. We just must be patient and try to keep everyone in as good shape as possible until that little machine comes along.

I continue, "Other very active research is going on in the field of prevention and treatment of complications. The Diabetes Control and Complications Trial, known as the DCCT, has recently shown us that good blood glucose control can prevent or delay complications that strike the eyes, the kidney, and the nerves. It is believed that keeping the hemoglobin A1c in an excellent range can do lots for prevention. Blindness need not be in the future for people with diabetes. Certainly, the laser therapy, which you heard about last night, is encouraging for those who do develop problems.

"We also know now that it's very important to screen and follow blood pressures. Early treatment of high blood pressure and early treatment for kidney disease may slow the progression of damage. Researchers are getting closer to the prevention of both the disease and its complications." I hope that gives the optimistic

197

viewpoint I truly believe. It's how long will it take that's the big question.

"So our job is to keep our children as healthy as possible until that time," states Lisa. The others agree and appear to be pleased about the research news.

Of course, we all want "the cure" as soon as possible. It's hard to be patient. But we have no choice but to work with what we have. My job is to stay up to date on the current treatments and be in tune with any significant advances. I like to think I can refer my patients to anywhere in the country for the latest protocols if they want to be involved. But I also like to think it's my job to be a cautious, objective advisor to families who may become overenthusiastic about some of the glorified "treatments" that occasionally appear in lay press.

I add, "The American Diabetes Association's magazine *Diabetes Forecast* has a research issue yearly, which is a good source of up-to-date information on the progress of some of these studies. Lots of research is going on and that, to me, is very exciting. I really enjoy going to research meetings and keeping abreast. But the progress is always slower than we'd like. I guarantee you when a better treatment is found, you'll hear about it."

"Call me, night or day, Doc," says Darryl. The group laughs nervously. It's painfully obvious that's what everyone wants. And believe me, all diabetes professionals would like to have the opportunity to make that phone call.

The first part of the morning has flown by. We have a few more important things to cover, but it's time for a break. I wonder how Pat and Heather are doing with the kids. They were planning to have them illustrate the kids diabetes book and then evaluate camp. Pat plans to have Eddy and Ginny play our "Diabetes Jeopardy Game" with the kids, while she and Heather join me for the next part of the morning.

The swinging doors open abruptly. Our two littlest campers, Emily and Little Lucy, run in. Both have gooey apple slices in their hands. Emily holds out a slice for her dad. Sam graciously accepts.

"You want some maw?" Emily says with her mouth stuffed.

"Em, honey, don't talk with your mouth full," instructs Pearl, softly. "Daddy was just coming out for his snack." Sam stands, and they walk out together. Actually, many adults don't have morning snacks, but Emily might not understand the difference. Sam can eat a small one, just to make Emily happy.

"Let's break for about 15 minutes, and then, when you return, we'll go over the tests." A few of the parents groan. They may have forgotten about the pre-test we gave on Sunday. But we haven't. After the re-test, we'll go over each question and discuss any problems. In the past it's been a good review and the parents have been quite pleased with their improvement.

Pat and I have always wanted to somehow scientifically evaluate the value of this camp. But to write an article for a scientific journal, or even submit an abstract to a national meeting, you must have statistics. Case histories and family comments don't scientifically prove our camp's worth. We need information that proves the parents and kids learn more about diabetes while they're here.

But that's not the most beneficial part of camp. It's the sharing and caring that goes on, along with the learning. We know we should contact all the former campers to see if, after several years, they still think this camp provided them with something lasting. But clinical research and paper writing take a lot of energy and time. And, luckily, I'm not on the academic track of having to publish or perish. Here in Maine I'm able to practice medicine, providing a worthwhile service, by caring for people. I'm relatively unencumbered by endless committee meetings, academic promotional hassles, and such, which are so prevalent at the large University Hospitals.

Still, I would like to see this family camp concept spread. One of our former campers, a Maine government health official who came here with his daughter and wife, said, "I believe every family with diabetes should have the opportunity to come to this camp." That was very flattering, but, of course, impossible. We can only take eight families at a time. Even if we worked for 10 weeks in the summer, that would only be 80 families. Hardly a dent. That's why other week-long camps need to be developed.

It makes me laugh to think of another great dad who was here from New York. He was a real promoter. He said we should bring this experience down to the City. I remember he claimed we could charge a lot more money for it down there. He was even willing to find the location and help us. We hesitated. For us, part of the magic of this week is the location. Everyone must be relaxed, not receiving faxed letters from their busy offices. The environment must lend itself to introspection. There must be opportunities for peaceful silence—serene moments to be with family members, away from the hustle of business and social commitments. It's got to be a vacation as well as an education.

"Joan, do you have the evaluation forms and the tests?" Pat's question immediately brings me back to the moment. But of course I have to take a few seconds to recall just where I left the pile of papers I carried over earlier this morning. By the look on Pat's face, I can tell she wonders why she gave them to me in the first place. But she says nothing.

"Um, I think they are . . . um . . . either . . . on the piano or in the telephone room." Thank goodness, they're on the piano. I have a habit of putting things down and then not remembering exactly where I've put them. Pat can usually find them, though. We have a standing joke. She's not to give me anything terribly important unless she first makes a copy. I won't lose the original, but I might just temporarily misplace it. I don't know what I'd do without her.

"How was your session with the kids?" I ask.

"It was a riot, especially the evaluation part. Tate has basically decided that he'll be back every year from now on. He wanted to reserve the same room for next year but requested that Eddy move upstairs, maybe into Ginny's room. And when he said that, Ginny blushed. Basically, the kids didn't have too many suggestions, except for more water slide time and maybe a swimming pool."

"Well, those sound like good suggestions. But somehow I don't think the Hersey Board will go for the pool idea. I'd like to suggest a tennis court. What do you think?"

"I think we'll have to stick with baseball and volleyball and some awesome kite flying. And the mud hike. Susan said she thought we should have a mud hike every day. And Cindy wants camp to last at least 12 more weeks. Nobody thought camp was too long. Tate said it should be a week because he didn't think people could pack enough clothes for two weeks."

"Sounds like the kids had plenty of comments. They really have gotten to be good friends."

"They had some curious ideas about what they thought camp was going to be like. Kevin thought we'd all be on a diet with lots of carrots and stuff. He's been pleasantly surprised by the great food. He also thought there would be boring lectures all day. I'd say he was the most pleased with the daily mixture of learning and fun."

"And eating," I add.

"And Abigail thought we'd all be in little cabins with out-houses. Becky said she thought it was going to be just a plain house with nine rooms, a kitchen and living room. They all like going over to the French House for meals and having the huge game room here with the ping-pong and pool tables."

"So we got a pretty good evaluation from the kids at least."

"Yeah, and Becky even said she might want to return some day as a counselor." Pat raises her eyebrows.

"That's great. She can have something positive to think of when she thinks of her diabetes. And that could just be the miracle. You never know." Pat and I exchange a few more thoughts.

As the parents return to the meeting room, Pat and I hand out the exams. "If you'll just answer the ones on the test that are circled. Those are the ones that you missed the first time around. Then we'll go over each question. Do you all have pencils?" Pat asks. Brent passes the box of pencils. Sam, who missed quite a few answers the first time around, concentrates. His attitude has changed so much.

I know Emily is happier with this change in her father. Certainly Pearl will now have some help. We see changes like this at camp, but wonder how long they will last at home. At least with Sam and Emily, we'll be seeing them again.

"Heather, is number 26 a trick question?" Marjorie asks.

"Marj, do you think we'd do something like that? Of course it is. We wouldn't want you to get them all right. Otherwise, you wouldn't need us to teach this class." Heather and Marjorie have taken to kidding each other. I recall how frustrated Heather was with Marjorie and her husband at the beginning of the week. But both Brent and Marjorie have relaxed and warmed up to the group. It sometimes takes longer for the out-of-staters, especially the more reserved and guarded metropolitan types, to relax and feel welcome. One year it was Thursday before the group meshed. But eventually, it did.

The rest of the morning we review the answers. Most of the questions are pretty basic. Several questions check on vocabulary to be sure all the parents know the medical terms for high blood sugar (hyperglycemia), low blood sugar (hypoglycemia), rebound (a high blood sugar level following a low blood sugar), glucagon (a hormone that will raise blood sugar by stimulating the liver to release sugar) and honeymoon period (time after diagnosis when insulin requirements are low). Other questions relate to symptoms the parents can see in their child. They all admit to being confused at times by the occasional similarity in irritability seen in some kids with both high and low blood sugar.

Heather reviews the answers about the basic food groups, as well as some on artificial sweeteners and the new fat substitutes.

"Heather," Brent asks, "what is the percentage of fat that we should be aiming for in our diet? I guessed less than 10 percent."

"The American Diabetes Association currently recommends less than 30 percent of calories from fat. Unsaturated fats, those in vegetable oils or margarine, are recommended over saturated fat, those from meat and dairy products."

The fathers have learned about meal planning. Food questions are usually the toughest for fathers, because most are just not involved in the planning or cooking of the meals for their kids.

"I get the feeling you're not totally convinced these new fat substitutes are going to be the miracle," Mark comments.

"I guess I believe in moderation. It wouldn't be desirable to remove all fat from our diet. Fats are necessary for vitamin absorption, and they provide a good source of energy, too. Besides, most of the kids with diabetes are not overweight, unlike so many of the people with Type II diabetes. These fat substitutes may be of bigger use for obese people.

"It's also important to be aware that some of the fat substitutes are made from protein. Researchers think it's important to watch the amount of protein that folks with diabetes eat. Too much protein can put a strain on the kidneys. So we need to be careful and use moderation with these new products. I'm sure there'll be a role for these fat substitutes, just as there's a place for artificial sweeteners, but you need to look at the whole picture and stay informed about the beneficial and harmful effects of these dietary manipulations."

"Do you have a 'hot line' we can dial for diet information?" Nancy asks, with a smile.

"Nancy, that's a great idea," Pat says. "We'll set that up for Heather at the hospital. What should we call it, 'Dial-a-Diet Dialogue'."

"No, seriously, there are so many new products and claims in magazines and on TV that I find it impossible to figure it all out. It would be great to be able to get the truth," Marjorie adds.

"I find the *Diabetes Forecast* magazine pretty up to date on this type of information," Lucy comments.

"Yes, it does have many helpful articles, and I'd be delighted to have you call me if questions arise. And we cover nutrition in our diabetes clinics, if any of you will be able to come next fall," Heather says.

Pearl jumps in. "Emily, Sam, and I are coming, for sure."

"Great!" Pat replies.

"I think we've gone over all the questions. Any other subjects on your minds?" There is a long pause. No more questions. It's been a pretty solid hour and a half of review and learning.

Pat hands out the evaluation forms. We do this mostly to get constructive criticism and any good hints for future years. By the end of the week we can pretty well feel what everyone thinks, but again for documentation we ask them to evaluate both the facilities and the program. Is there too much teaching or not enough? Was there enough free time or too much. Did you enjoy the guests, like Tim Rogers and Dr. Takash and Paul? Were your children's needs met? Were yours? And what did you get out of camp that you didn't expect? What did you like the best? The least? Then we ask for any other comments and suggestions.

"If you would just take some time now or after lunch to fill these out, we'd really appreciate it. Please, be honest. We really would like to hear any criticisms you have so we can continue to improve our program. Just hand them back before tonight, if possible."

Heather, Pat, and I leave the room to give the parents some privacy and to check on the kids. It's is 11:45, and they're all still playing the Jeopardy game. Emily and Little Lucy are missing, as is Ginny. Pat suggests that Eddy end the game so we can check blood sugars. With the mention of lunch, the game quickly ends. Peter, Becky, Susan, Jeff, and Kevin all go to the table for testing. Pat reminds them to wash their hands first. Emily and Little Lucy come down the stairs with Ginny, who tells me she's been helping the little girls with their act for tonight. But she gives me no clue what their act is.

Editor's note: Research information included in this chapter has been updated through December 1995.

How You Play the Game

During rest hour Pat, Heather, and I work hard to perfect (well, *nearly*) our class acts. We make out the awards for tonight and only have three campers we haven't matched up with an appropriate award. But this afternoon's events may give us our inspiration.

It's warmed up nicely. Another sunny day, and Penobscot Bay, world famous for great sailing, is dotted with sailboats. We're so lucky to have it in our own backyard.

Back at the main lodge, Eddy says all is ready. He and Ginny have gathered the props for the games: a dozen eggs, four tablespoons, lots of blindfolds, and various purses, hats, skirts, and shirts for the costume race. Tate rings the bell, and we all gather at the baseball diamond for the start of the field day games.

Pat announces the opening game, called "Animal Farm." In a large circle, everyone is first blindfolded and then counts off—one, two, three, four. This repeats all the way around the circle. All the ones are to be cows, the twos are dogs, threes, sheep, and fours, cats. We separate the blindfolded campers and spread them out all over the baseball field. Then, at the signal, the animals are to find their litter mates by loudly making their sound and carefully advancing in the direction of similar sound. The few observers have the most fun, watching and listening as the moo-moos, bow-wows, meow-meows, and baa-baas find each other. Sam, Brent, Darryl, and Mark—these grown men wander with their arms extended, chuckling together. Only in Maine, only at Camp Kee-to-Kin.

Another fun game is Giants, Elves, and Wizards. It's similar to the old hand game of scissors, paper, and rock. The giants chase the elves, the elves chase the wizards, and the wizards chase the giants. This game takes concentration. But the little kids delight in running away from the enemy, back to their line of safety. Even though she's a mighty slow runner, Lydia enjoys this game. If she is being chased, all the kids on the other side capture her. She makes quite a production out of being captured, much to the delight of Tate and some of the other boys. Lucy watches this game from the sidelines, but cheers everyone on.

For the egg tossing contest, Lucy and Lydia join forces. Lucy is so petite and Lydia so large. But both know how to throw and catch an egg. Twice the egg bounces on the ground, but it doesn't break. The grass is soft. Kevin accuses his mother of having a hard boiled egg. In the end, after everyone else's egg has broken, Lucy and Lydia are still tossing it. On the last throw to Lydia the egg lands in her hands and smashes. She laughs, as the yolk and egg white drip through her fingers.

The games go on. The fun knot game gets the adults really giggling. Teamwork definitely comes into play, as this enmeshed group, with hands linked to other hands, try to unwind by going over, under, and around each other. The kids perform their maneuvers well, getting a greater kick out of watching their parents stretch and laugh their way to freedom.

This is a time to let out the child in you. We all have that child in there, but many people are afraid to let it out, to be free from the restraints of grown-up rules. Sometimes we're too serious, too concerned, too burdened.

Pat gives instructions for the last event. "For our final game we'll have a costume race. Sam, Mark, Darryl, and Brent will be the starters. Form four lines, one behind each starter." The group divides up fairly evenly into four groups. "The object is to put on the costume (which includes purse, hat, shirt, pants, or skirt), run to the imaginary line where Heather is, run back, undress, and the next member dresses and runs down and back. Winners get to go down the water slide first."

Jeff jumps up and down. He's been asking all day about the water slide. Even Little Lucy wants to try it again. And today with this warm weather, there shouldn't be too many blue lips.

"On your mark, get set, go!" Pat hollers. The four men quickly try to dress. Sam throws the skirt over his head, but it won't come down over his large shoulders, he leaves it draped there, and clutching his purse, he dashes off with his other hand holding the cowboy hat on his head. Darryl and Mark are not far behind. Brent, with large flowery Bermuda shorts, laughs so hard, he can hardly pick up his pocketbook. What a sight! The kids howl, the mothers giggle. Each camper gets a turn. Even Lucy tries this final game. She's a quick dresser and limps down the field. Nancy, who is racing against Lucy, is laughing so hard that she loses her hat and must run back to fetch it. As they cross the finish line, Lucy and Nancy get a big round of applause.

"Snacks are up on the porch. Be sure to eat a good one if you've exercised hard during the games and if you're planning to do the water slide," says Heather. The kids charge up the hill, as the rest of us gather the props and more slowly stroll up to the lodge.

"Where did you learn all those games?" Pearl asks.

"Oh, we've collected them over the years," I reply.

"I haven't laughed so much in a long time," she adds. I put my arm around her, and we hike up the hill.

Again the water slide is popular. Heather assures me that all the kids had juice and some cheese and crackers. Pat checks Susan's blood sugar before she goes to slide. It's just fine. We don't want another reaction. She's done well for the last few days since we decreased her insulin dosage. Brent and Marjorie are delighted with the change in their daughter. Through her purple-rimmed glasses, her eyes now sparkle.

As the kids and a few courageous parents slide down the side of the hill, Ginny and I bring over the picnic supplies from the French House. Tonight is the cook's night off, so we have a picnic at the lodge. Darryl volunteers to start the charcoal fire and Sam offers him a hand. Neither look keen to try the water slide. On our second trip over with the food, I notice Emily trying to pull her father toward the slide. Jeff appears to be reminding Sam that he had agreed to it this morning. I'm amazed that Emily has gone down, but as I approach the slide, Pat tells me that Little Lucy and Emily went down together, giving each other moral support.

At the bottom both grinned from ear to ear. And now Emily wants her father to go down with her, just as Mark did at first with Little Lucy. Sam puts up a small battle. Darryl assures him the charcoal will be fine. Eventually, he gives in, sliding down with Emily between his legs, and Jeff and Kyle riding behind. At the bottom he stands, picks up his daughter, and gives the victory sign. Pearl applauds from above as the four charge up the hill, probably to do it again.

Marjorie, Nancy, and Lisa, sitting on rocking chairs on the porch, watch the sailboats. The evening is glorious. A warm, gentle breeze brushes across their faces. Each looks so relaxed. The two out-of-staters soak up their last evening in Maine. Pennsylvania and Ohio are a far cry from the shores of Penobscot Bay and the grassy fields of Hersey Retreat.

I overhear them talking. "Well, you'll just have to come back and visit us," Lisa says to them both. "I know my kids would love to see Susan, Tate, and Becky again. We could show you all around Bar Harbor and Acadia. The view from Cadillac Mountain is great."

"I remember driving up there with Brent once. I think it was our second date," Marjorie adds.

"Darryl and I will be back for sure. We're going to take a cruise next year on one of the schooners." Nancy's already dreaming of it.

"Dr. MacCracken, I think the coals are ready for the burgers and dogs." Darryl prepares the charcoal bed, and the time for cooking is at hand. Lydia, who has been talking with Ginny and Heather, volunteers to be in charge of the buns. As the aroma of freshly grilled burgers spreads, the water sliders cease their activities, dry off, check their blood sugars, and take their pre-supper insulin. Pat gives the kids with diabetes a helping hand, but most of them know the ropes by now. Even Emily pricks her own finger now. A giant step from the first day of crying.

The charcoal-broiled burgers and hot dogs are a big hit, as are the special Maine baked beans and the garden fresh salad. Everyone mingles. Peter, Jeff, Kyle, Susan, and Abigail perch on the porch railing, talking rapidly as they eat. Becky's portable compact disc player provides music for the three girls (Becky, Ginny, and Cindy), who sit off near the sandbox. Ginny has done a great job with these two girls. Munching their burgers between points, Eddy and Kevin continue the challenge ping-pong match. Kevin may have met his match.

"Joan," Lydia says, "I sure hope we can come back next year. Kevin and Cindy really like it here. And it's been a good break for me, too."

I'm sure this has been a good break for them all. Their cramped little mobile home as well as the tension of Kevin's manipulations and hospitalizations offer little space for enjoyment.

"Wait here a minute," she says. Stuffing her final bite of hot dog bun into her mouth, she dashes into the lodge and disappears up the stairs.

Brent comes over to speak with me. "So when do you plan to visit us in Philadelphia? We have to get in a squash game, you know."

"Well, I'll be down for my twenty-fifth reunion from medical school in a few years. I'll be sure to look you up when I get in town— that is, if you're still there then. Your wife's dreaming of a Maine cottage in Blue Hill to retire to early." I smile.

"Sounds nice, but I'm afraid I've got a few more kids to put through college before I can retire."

"Yeah, I know what you mean."

Kevin and Lydia come out of the lodge. She is carrying a plastic bag, the one Lou gave her when he came to visit. Lydia gets Cindy to join them. Then she grabs Heather and Pat and brings them over to me.

Lydia, now embarrassed to speak, nudges her son. Kevin starts, "My mom wants me to tell you that we've all had a great time, and we thought you guys might like these."

His mother pulls out one figurine at a time, giving Heather, Pat, and me each one. We all grin. These are the products of Lydia's labors. She makes these funny looking people out of lobster shells. Many gift shops along the coast sell figures similar to these. The red hard shells and claws of the cooked lobster form the head and body of the figure. Heather's is a fisherman. A long pole stands between his hands (claws). Pat's looks like a washerwoman, and mine, which I like the best, is a lobsterwoman with a lobsterbaby on her lap. These are very cleverly made. The expressions on the faces are priceless.

"Thank you so much," I say, as I give Kevin, Cindy, and Lydia hugs. Pat and Heather do the same. These are the indescribable rewards.

"Lydia, these are fantastic! You have quite a knack for making these appear so real," Pat adds.

"Mom can make ten in one day," Kevin brags proudly. "She won the Port Clyde lobster figurine contest two years ago."

"Well, I can see why," Heather comments. All the kids crowd around to look at our new gifts. Darryl and Nancy are fascinated by these strange creatures, never seen in Ohio.

"Where we come from, the claws just go in the garbage."

"Well, us Mainers don't liken to waste nothing, ah-yup!" Mark says in his heavy Maine accent. We all laugh.

The strawberry Jello cubes are perfect for dessert. You just pick them up and plop them in your mouth. A fun, low-calorie delight. Pat comments, "After dessert, let's all pick up. There's a big trash bag over by the door. We'll start the talent show at 7 o'clock."

Discovering
Our Talents

Our stage is set. The benches face the front, and a few chairs line the sides. Pat will use a big pad of paper, held up by an easel, to announce the acts. The front sheet reads, "The 10th Annual Camp Kee-to-Kin No Talent, Some Talent, Great Talent Show." The kids grab the front row seats.

Just before 7 o'clock, Steve arrives. His family is happy to see him again, and the other campers greet him too. Obviously, he's not considered a stranger here. Occasionally, in the past we've had outsiders come for the talent show, and it hasn't worked.

Everyone feels pretty close by Friday night. And some folks are willing to perform within this new extended family, but if strangers or even uninvolved family members arrive, the campers' inhibitions return. But tonight, Steve is part of the family, even though he could only join us for the campfire on Wednesday night.

Becky sets her CD player on top of the piano and tucks her clarinet in behind. She winks at me, as she walks toward her father, who is saving her a seat. The commotion of prop preparation and final organization dies down.

Pat begins. "Welcome, ladies, gentlemen, and kids of all ages. Tonight, you will have the opportunity to see the Camp Kee-to-Kin No Talent, Some Talent, Great Talent Show." Pat loves to ham things up. "Many of these acts have never been seen before. Most will never be seen again." The crowd laughs. "So, to start things off, our First Act will be the 'Hersey Retreat Tooters'."

Wearing matching Hersey Retreat T-shirts, Heather, Pat and I gather up front with our recorders. "One, two, three," Pat starts us off. And away we go, playing our tunes in a round. Pat swings her head back and forth, I tap my foot, and Heather leans forward to see the cue card. Amazingly, we end at approximately the same time and in harmony. We bow, as the audience rewards the first act with their applause. We've successfully broken the ice.

"Thank you," Pat says. Our next act will be Camp Kee-to-Kin's own Bobby McFerrin with his two assistants, singing that famous hit tune, 'Don't Worry, Be Happy'." Eddy comes onstage with a colorful paisley shirt and his fluorescent shorts. He has darkened in a beard and mustache. Ginny and Becky, in colorful outfits, stand over by the piano. Becky turns on the tape recorder, and the familiar tune starts up. Eddy lip-syncs the words, as the girls join in for the chorus.

> *"Here's a little song I wrote.*
> *You might want to sing it note for note,*
> *Don't worry, be happy.*
> *In every life we have some trouble,*
> *But when you worry, you make it double,*
> *Don't worry, be happy . . . ."*

As the song goes along, all the campers join in on the chorus. Eddy has marvelous hand movements, and he has learned the words perfectly; he's in sync. Repeating the chorus line, Eddy and his girls stroll out the swinging doors. We all clap. The three return, and remind me that they got the idea from our Ellsworth trip. I congratulate them on a great rendition.

And the acts roll on. The kids put on their puppet show, which they've practiced only once or twice. Abigail plays a great nurse, and Tate acts out quite a reaction. Hidden behind the puppet stage, the children are even less inhibited than usual. Next, Becky plays a beautiful melody on her clarinet, "Pacobel Canon," I think. Nancy and Darryl grin with pride. Emily and Little Lucy, with some coaxing, go next with the hand game, "A Sailor Went to Sea, You See." Ginny helps sing the song with them, and for five and four year olds, both do remarkably well. Pearl and Sam beam. Their little Emily has come out of her shell, all right.

"I'm not exactly sure what the next act is all about, but the participants will be Jeff, Kyle, and their mother, Lucy, and they've titled this act, 'Seven Days of Camp'." The two boys stand next to their mother, who holds a sheet of paper out in front of them.

Lucy says, "The boys helped me write this song, and it's in honor of the Camp Kee-to-Kin staff. They begin,

On the first day of camp, my counselors gave to me,
    a blood glucose testing machine.
On the second day of camp my counselors gave to me,
    two Ketostix and a blood glucose testing machine."

The song goes to seven days (instead of the twelve days of Christmas) and ends like this:

"Seven cotton swabs, six lancets, five syringes,
four fruit exchanges, three glucose tabs, two ketostix,
and a blood glucose testing machine."

Kyle and Jeff shake hands to congratulate themselves for getting through it. Steve, their dad, applauds loudly, as Eddy and I give loud whistles. A very clever creation.

"For our next act, Nancy and Marjorie have created their version of 'The Price is Right,' called 'The Calories are Right.' Abigail and

Susan will be their assistants." Both of these rather reserved women are animated tonight. Marjorie directs the two girls to begin the show with their song.

Swinging their arms back and forth, the two girls sing, "Radishes are beautiful, radishes are fine, I like radishes, I eat them all the time. I eat them for my supper, and I eat them for my lunch, if I haven't got to hurry, I'd eat them all at once." Then, after a few giggles, they add, "Welcome to 'The Calories are Right'."

Nancy says, "Now, we need two contestants from our studio audience. Our assistants will draw names out of the hat. And our first contestant is . . ." Abigail unfolds the paper and reads "Heather." Susan reads the other name, "Mark."

"Come on down," Marjorie and Nancy cry. Both contestants approach the table and two chairs. On the table are two white towels, each covering a bowl, one in front of each contestant. Paper napkins are ceremoniously draped around the contestants' necks. "To win a free vacation to Bangor, Maine, all expenses paid including two tickets to the oldest community symphony orchestra in the country, one of you must be the first to consume the 500 calories now placed in front of you. Are you ready?"

Heather and Mark are already laughing, but both prepare to start eating. Simultaneously, Nancy and Marjorie remove the towels and expose the calories. Heather bursts out laughing, holding up her bowl of what must be at least three hundred radishes. Mark is all smiles, as he shows his three chocolate cup cakes. He starts eating the first one slowly, as Heather eats three or four radishes and then pleads for some help from the audience. Everyone thinks this is a great joke on the camp nutritionist. I guess the dietary auction has returned to haunt Heather.

Pat wipes tears of laughter from her cheeks. Heather congratulates Marjorie and Nancy on a great joke. "And now, after he gets the chocolate off his face, Mark has agreed to tell us another Maine story. So, here in our own backyard, once again, we have Tim Sample's fill-in, 'Mainiac Mark.' In a very thick Maine accent Mark tells his traveling salesman story. Like a magician, he holds everyone's attention. And with the punch line, the adults all laugh, and a few of the older kids get it. The combination of the wonderful Maine accent and the silly story make me laugh, too.

"Next act, we meet," Pat flips the page on the easel, "Camp KTK's Karate Kid." Tate comes crashing through the swinging doors, wearing his official karate uniform. His father calls out the moves, as Tate very seriously performs these learned skills. It's amazing to see how much this little six year old knows. We give him a round of applause.

The acts are running smoothly, and it's fun to have surprise performances. "And now Nancy and Cindy will sing 'Climb Every Mountain' from *The Sound of Music*."

The group quiets down as Nancy settles in front of piano and plays the introduction. At first there is a little hesitation in her playing. I suspect it's been a while since she's performed in public. But when she begins to sing, her fingers flow across the keyboard, and the notes stream from her mouth and, I'd say, soul.

Standing by Nancy, Cindy looks out beyond the audience. She knows these words by heart. Their voices blend beautifully. There are a few teary eyes in the audience as Nancy and Cindy finish. It's so lovely several campers request an encore and Nancy and Cindy comply. A few of the campers quietly sing along. I look over at Pat. If camp were just for this one exhilarating moment, it would all be worth it.

As Cindy returns to her seat, Lydia gives her a big hug. I overhear her say, "That was so beautiful, Cin." And Kevin pats her on the back, like a very proud brother.

"I'm sure I speak for the entire group here that we think you two should continue to pursue your singing careers. That was just fantastic," Pat says. Becky's smile is worth a thousand words.

From the sublime to the ridiculous, the next act is our new song. Ginny introduces us, "And now for your continued entertainment, 'Chief Somogyi and the Rebounds'." Out in the hallway Pat, Heather, and I begin changing into our costumes. Realizing it will take a few moments, I ask Mark to tell one more short Maine story. He keeps the audience entertained as we strap on our feathers and beads.

Heather wraps up in a colorful blanket. With her black hair, now tied with a leather headband holding several paper feathers, she looks great. Pat and I wear beads and a single feather. The face paint helps set our scene.

We give Ginny the high sign, and she announces us again. This time, we appear. Heather sits on a table with her legs crossed and her head bowed, while Pat and I begin the chant, beating our wooden sticks together. We repeat again and again, "Lower your sugar, lower your sugar."

At an inspired moment, Heather throws back her head and lifts her arms to the sky, crying "Insulin, innn-sullll-in, innn-sull-in, into your fat." The chants continue, with Heather wailing out her cries.

Pat and I try to continue chanting, but whenever Heather erupts with her prayer, we can hardly contain ourselves. Luckily, the rest of the audience is laughing too. The final chant, Pat and I say, 'Camp Kee-to-Kin' over and over, and Heather cries out, "Families, families, families, that's where it's at." And with that we end. If, by now, the whole camp doesn't think we three are crazy, they probably never will.

Everyone's wild. This electrified atmosphere is exactly what the next group needs to perform. "For our last act before the awards, we have some guys who want to sing a song or two. In fact, they call themselves 'The Latin LaBamba Laddies'."

Becky starts up her tape player and the sound of castanets begins. With T-shirts on and the sleeves rolled up, Brent, Darryl, Mark, and Sam dance through the doors. Sam, with his Camels wrapped up in the left sleeve, and Brent, with his hair slicked back, definitely look like rock 'n roll sixties tough guys.

Darryl, wearing Susan's purple rimmed sunglasses, looks more like Elton John. And Mark's just one of the guys. Each try to lip-sync the Spanish words to the song, "LaBamba" as they hop up and down. Two of them keep a great beat. The other two keep trying. As the music fades, the audience yells and whistles their appreciation. The "LaBamba Laddies" take their bows. Mark's a total ham. These fathers are enjoying their own antics.

The next song, blaring out from the stereo tape deck, is "Get a Job." Brent holds up a microphone made from a stick with a tennis ball on top. He does a great job singing the words while the others coordinate their chorus, "Dip Dip, Dip, Dip, Boon, Boon, Boon, Get a Job." Another roar from the campers.

And when the final song, "Tequila" starts, the beat is just too powerful to resist. Pat grabs Eddy, and they begin to boogie. Following Pat's lead, Heather pulls Kevin into the group. Others start dancing at their seats. I lift Little Lucy and Emily onto the benches, and they wiggle to the music. The room is wild with dancing. Becky, who has turned up the volume some, has never looked happier.

After the final "Tequila," we all collapse in laughter and applause. The men take their seats, as everyone tells them how great they are. Ginny divulges that they practiced late into the night last night, and wouldn't let anyone in the room. Every year we're amazed by the campers. Such shy, withdrawn folks on Sunday now being so silly and chuckling at themselves. Certainly, we all know the world could use more laughter and frivolity.

"Well, that was a fabulous ending to our show. You men may have discovered a new career. You must promise to continue with your new-found talents. Thanks for all the wonderful acts. This was a great show." We clap again. Brent asks Marjorie to snap a shot of the rock group.

As soon as Pat jots down a few additional notes, she starts the awards. "Some of you have asked me how we measure success of camp. Well, each camp is different. Each of you bring to it something special. All of the years have been unique. None better or best. All are wonderful, all are special. And they are all these things because of you.

"This year, you can be especially proud of your children, who have been well-behaved, cooperative, helpful, creative, well-mannered, and tolerant. And that is a credit to all of you. And it's encouraging to us to see families work and play hard together. It's also very exciting to see total strangers become, in one week, a big close family. We know you come with fears, taking some big risks, since some of you don't even know us." A few quips filter up from the friendly audience. "And we appreciate your willingness to be with us and to be so caring for each other. We've seen new things happen this week, and using these observations we'd like to give out our awards.

"First, we'd like to thank our two counselors. Ginny, Eddy, come on up here." Everyone claps as they gather around Pat. "You two have been a great addition to our camp this year. Eddy wanted to come back after being away for seven years. He's been an open and honest source of feelings and information for all of us, and I know he has learned a few things here from you, too." He nods as he puts his arm around Pat. "And we hope he'll consider coming back next year. He was Father Eddy at the costume party, ran a mean hundred yard dash carrying a bowl of Cheerios for Susan one night, and surprised us all with his Bobby McFerrin singing. He's not only a good role model, but also a great model, loaning us his marvelous physique for our injection sites demonstration." Eddy blushes.

Pat continues, "He's one special and sensitive guy, and we give him the Camp KTK Mr. Goodbody Award." All the kids shout and clap. He's well loved by everyone. "And, in addition, we have two tickets for him to see his favorite Boston Red Sox at Fenway Park next month." Eddy gives Pat a big hug, and then comes over and gives me one, too.

"Now, Ginny is a marvel. I never had to ask her to do anything. She was always five minutes ahead of my request and seemed to know when one of the kids needed some special attention. She told Dr. MacCracken just yesterday that she wished she had two little sisters like Emily and Little Lucy. Ginny has been a constant source of encouragement. She's frank, determined, and has one of the most positive outlooks that I've seen. We'd love to get her back next year, but I bet she has big plans for future summers. All I can say is, look out Boston, look out Washington, here she comes. Ginny, we give you the 'Go for the Gold' Award."

Again, boisterous applause. I walk over to her and add jokingly, "Because I've heard say that the only good lawyer is a judge, we have for you an official gavel." She laughs as I give her the gift. There's little doubt in my mind that Ginny will make a great lawyer, and who knows she might even be a Maine senator or our first woman President."

Pat goes on. "We have some really special kids here this year. For the little kids, our educational sessions can be pretty boring. But this little girl was quiet and kept herself entertained. She got to meet her first real live clowns this week, and she conquered her initial fear of going down the water slide. She's an adorable kid, whom we've all grown to love. At four years old Lucy gets the 'Best Little Sister' Award." She hops off her mother's lap, and runs up to Pat, who hands her the blue ribbon award. Pat gives her a little kiss on the cheek, and Lucy runs back to her mom.

"This little guy, well, he isn't so little, is sensitive and concerned. He loves playing with his brother and finds diabetes inconvenient, because it interrupts their playing time. He's a whiz at Legos." Now, everyone knows whom she is talking about. "Kyle has learned a lot about diabetes and even gave himself an injection to see how it feels, and he gets the 'Concerned, Sensitive, and Playful Big Brother' Award." Kyle proudly comes up to claim his award, as everyone cheers. Steve and Lucy beam.

"Way to go, Kyle!" shouts Peter.

Pat continues to hand out the awards. She has a way of making everyone feel really special about themselves. And it isn't that hard, because some big changes can be seen at camp. But the way she does it, by saying several positive things, before giving perhaps a humorous award, makes the evening. Susan receives the "Purple Passion" Award and Becky, who has changed the most, receives the "It's All Right, Baby" award. She whispers, "thanks" to me as she walks by. Peter is the "Most Athletic" camper. He's proud of that. And Kevin, because of his outlandish bathing suit costume, wins the "Miss Camp Kee-to-kin Award." He's able to laugh at that one. Lydia and Cindy enjoy the chuckle, too.

"This young woman," Pat continues, "may just replace me some day. She listens to everything we say about diabetes. She's concerned about her big brother and always wants to help. At the young age of eight, Abigail deserves the 'Honorary Camp KTK Registered Nursing' Award. And Ginny helped us make a special nurse's hat for her." Ginny uses a few bobby pins to fix the RN hat on Abigail's head. She looks adorable. Her father and mother both stand and clap for her accomplishment. Brent snaps a shot.

"That a way, Sis," says Peter.

"The next kid is determined in many ways. He plays hard and is always on the go. I think he played more pool games this week than anyone. He knows lots about diabetes and came to camp determined to learn to draw up and give himself his own shot. That's not such an easy task at seven years old, but he did it. Jeff wants to help his mom any way he can. And we're all very proud of him for that. He and his brother also did a pretty good job at impersonating the ladies. Tonight, Jeff gets the 'I Can Do It Independence' Award."

Steve wipes a cheerful tear off of his wife's cheek. They both have much to be proud of. And we're so thankful they came to camp.

"Our oldest child, well, I better call her our teenager, came to camp not knowing what to expect. Neither did her mother or brother, for that matter. First, she found Becky and Ginny as sidekicks. And then she found Nancy, as a kindred spirit in song. She's a talented kid. She's caring and concerned about her brother's health. We know she is going to get somewhere with her beautiful voice. She gets the 'Glorious Songbird' Award."

Cindy has her hair tied back with a kerchief. Her eyes twinkle as she goes up to Pat, who gives her a great big hug. This is a changed kid. On that very first day, Cindy could barely lift her eyes off the floor, and her stringy hair covered her face. Nancy, without a doubt, has sparked an ember of hope. I hope we can nurture that flame. Maybe, just maybe, her mother will be able to appreciate her more and give her some very needed attention.

No one seems restless. They're amazingly quiet, listening to Pat. Tate, standing next to his father, whispers in his ear. He must know that it's almost his turn.

"This little kid," Pat says, and Tate starts to smile, "has changed a lot here at camp. In the beginning she was very shy and would hardly speak. She remembers how frightened she was of those old finger sticks. And I'm sure her grandmother never thought her granddaughter would go down the water slide. But Emily surprised us all. Now she does her own finger sticks; in fact, she prefers to do it herself now. And she doesn't even wince. And we all saw her go down that water slide this afternoon. I think she did it two times."

"Three times!" Jeff cries out.

"Well, three times she did it. She's made lots of friends this week, and I don't know what Little Lucy is going to do without her. And Emily loves rabbits. Everyone's met Inky this week, too. So to Emily and Inky, we give the 'Bunny Phoo-Phoo' Award."

Carrying Inky, Emily rushes up to Pat, who gives her the official award and a kiss. Then Emily turns and runs over to me with those little arms outstretched. I give her a big squeeze. I'll will miss this kid especially.

"And our final kid award goes to a live wire, a dynamo on two legs. This young man hit Hersey Retreat like a tornado. If he's not riding his bike, he's swinging on the tire or practicing his karate. He's climbed Blue Hill and splashed in the Atlantic Ocean. He tells me he wants to move to Maine now and not wait until his parents retire. I'm sure our state would not be the same with him. But we'll take him."

Tate, who has been very patiently waiting for this award, gets the 'Boundless Energy and Enthusiasm Plus' Award. He gets a round of applause. As he walks back to his seat, Tate can't resist giving Eddy a little punch.

"And we have great parents here, too. This year you've all jelled together. You've supported one another and been there with encouraging words. We all know that having a child with diabetes is tough. But after this week, we hope it will be just a little bit easier." Pat gives out awards to Lydia, Lisa, and Marjorie. Brent gets the "Ansel Adams Photography" Award and seems pleased.

She continues, "This couple also came to us from away—on a

leap of faith." I suppose Pat really means in search of a miracle, but that's a bit too heavy to mention. "They decided to drive all the way to Maine to experience our camp. We now know that Nancy needs to keep using her gorgeous voice, perhaps picking up her singing career again. And Darryl showed a lot of courage when he admitted that he's probably been running away from diabetes. Here at camp he's learned to face Becky's diabetes, and now he can provide more support to both Becky and Nancy. And together Nancy and Darryl have fallen in love with Maine, so we know we'll see them again. Tonight, both receive Camp Kee-to-Kin's 'Honorary Mainer' Awards."

They go up together to collect their ribbons. Eddy, who has had many long conversations with Darryl, cheers. Becky can't help but notice that her parents are holding hands as they walk up. I always get choked up when a change like this occurs. Once we had a mother and son who would hardly speak to each other on their arrival. All that changed in a week.

"This next lady is very special. She had two good reasons to come to camp, for her son and her granddaughter. She has the warmest heart around. I'm sure everyone would love to have such a loving grandmother as Pearl. We can't say enough about her determination to learn. Personally, I'm glad she stopped off at Hersey Retreat before going all the way to Boston for help. We are very thankful that she had her birthday this week so we could all help her celebrate. Pearl, you get the 'Most Knowledgeable and Loving Grandmother' Award. The campers cheer and hoot. Emily and Little Lucy jump up and down. Pearl hugs Pat, then me, then Heather, and then almost everybody else, as she returns to her seat.

Pat takes a deep breath. She's doing fine. "This dad has experienced just about everything here at camp. He was first adult down the water slide, he got a little muddy, and then quite wet on the mud hike. He entertains us with his great Maine stories. But besides all this, he's a very supportive husband and father. He's been willing to fly kites, play ping-pong, and read bedtime stories. His dish washing abilities are a bit limited." Everyone laughs, knowing he hates the short sink. "But besides that, he has been a great guy to have around. None of us will forget his Downeast accent. So Mark, you deserve the 'Say It Like It Is, Ah-yup! Storyteller' Award." It would be great to always have a special father like this around.

The camaraderie in the room is catching. Everyone wants everyone to feel good. Your basic mutual admiration society. My husband always tells me that each year it's almost like I've been through a religious experience. I don't know about that, but as the week draws quickly to a close, I sense the special bond. No one outside these doors can understand. I'm sure other small encounter groups go through this bonding. More people should try it.

Pat has two more awards to go. She holds up the next ribbon and pauses a moment to arrange her thoughts. All she has are a few notes or key words. The rest of her speech is spontaneous and straight from the heart. "This camper wasn't too sure he wanted to be here. In fact, I think, he contemplated leaving. Somehow, though, he decided to stay, and we're all glad he did. He knows two sides of diabetes, his own and his daughter's, and he has taught us all a lot." I can't help but look over at Becky. He certainly helped her. Pat goes on. "Those of us who were at the fort learned just how strong he is. And so for our strong hero of Fort Knox, we award Sam with this year's 'Paul Bunyan' award. Jeff, why don't you come up and give it to him?"

Jeff leaps up to beat Sam to the front of the room. He does. Jeff turns and hands the award to his new friend, Sam. They both shake. Sam shyly thanks Pat, and nods, smiling at me. No hugs are exchanged. That starless Monday night flashes before me, and I'm so glad I tried.

"This last lady is by no means last. The old saying 'last but not least' fits well. She has two little boys who love her lots and a very supportive husband who, luckily, could join us tonight. We've called her 'Big Lucy' most of the week. And though she is small in size, she is definitely big in spirit and courage. She joined us on the mud hike and in the dark caves of the fort. She tosses an egg better than anyone I've ever seen. Lucy, you have won our respect and love, and for you we have the 'Most Enthusiastic Parent' Award. As she rather slowly rises

223

to walk to the front, the entire group stands and claps for her. This lady is just plain super. Within that petit and somewhat frail body is a strong will and a dynamic personality. Everyone here will take home some lessons learned from Lucy. Of course, being the emotional slob that I am, I have to wipe away a few tears to see her accept her ribbon. And I'm quite sure I'm not the only one needing a Kleenex, either.

Pat comes over to Heather and me. "Well, are you guys up to the last act? I'm exhausted."

"You did a great job," I say softly.

"Sure, let's do it!" Heather says. "I'll make the announcement, you go out and get ready. Pat and I walk out the swinging doors. Heather gets the group's attention. We can hear her announce the final act, "The One and Only Camp Kee-to-Kin Andrew Sisters." She comes out and puts on her painter's hat. We three match—green Hersey Retreat T-shirts and white hats.

To the tune of "Oh, We Ain't Got a Barrel of Money" or better known as "Side by Side," we dance back into the room. After the slapping of our thighs to a catchy rhythm, we start the song:

Oh, it's the tenth great year that we have been
Right down here at Kee-to-Kin.
 With friends from away,
Buckeye and P.A.
Drive, Drive, Drive
(We do the thigh slapping routine and then shift places)

Water slide and the beach walk,
Education and small talk,
The lights, they went out,
But we didn't pout,
Flash, Flash, Flash
(More thigh slapping and rotation of places)

Ed returned after seven years
He helped us conquer our fears,
The counselors were neat,
At Hersey Retreat,
Thanks, thanks, thanks

Through all kinds of feelings
Who cares if we shed a tear,
Just as long as we share together,
And lend each other an ear.

Well, we'll all have our memories as we part,
Of fine friends, good food, and a new start,
We sure had great fun,
But now that it's done,
Bye, Bye, Bye
(We wave our hats and strut out the door,
      returning with the refrain)
We sure had great fun,
But now that it's done,
Bye, Bye, Bye.

We repeat the refrain once more as the audience applauds loudly. As we exit the last time, we stay out for awhile, and then finally go back in again. The show's over. The day's a success, and we're all exhausted.

Brent and Marjorie call for attention one last time. Brent says, "We just want to thank you three for a great week and give each of you one of these special cards that we have all signed and a flower from all of us. While Little Lucy, Emily, and Peter distribute the carnations, Abigail, Susan, and Tate give out the home-made cards. Eddy leads the groups in a cheer.

Pat, Heather, and I thank everyone for their thoughtfulness. Single red carnations, what a pleasant surprise. It feels so good to be appreciated.

The campers want to watch the talent show on video. While Heather starts up the popcorn machine, Eddy sets up the TV monitor and VCR. Pat and I help the kids do their blood sugars and record them on their charts. I'll keep the charts and send letters describing any changes that we have made to the campers' doctors. Tonight most of the kids are running a bit higher than their usual. I'd guess it's the excitement of the evening.

All the campers talk to one another. Six days and six nights together. Tomorrow these families will all go their separate ways. Some may never see each other again. Tonight the sharing continues. Spontaneously, the parents begin exchanging addresses and discussing plans for reunions or just casual get-togethers.

After the video has been played, Pat, Heather, and I say our good nights. Back in the cabin we open a bottle of wine that has been sitting on the shelf all week. We toast to each other and to a few good days of solitude we each plan to take before returning to our hospital work. We each know this one week of the year, though it may be intense, gives us new insights into diabetes and family interactions. Here we listen, we learn, and we grow.

Good-byes and Amens

"Joan, are you going to get up today?" Pat whispers from the door. I open my eyes, check my clock, and groan. Rarely do I ever oversleep. But there's no doubt I was about to. Dreams were floating by at a rapid pace.

"My alarm didn't go off. I must've needed a few extra winks."

"Well, I'll meet you over there." She turns and leaves.

I dress slowly. There's no rush. Everyone will be packing. Darryl will be trying to get off early. They're driving to Great Barrington, Massachusetts, a good half way point on their trip back to Ohio. I wonder if Nancy and Darryl feel they found their miracle. At least they are all three talking now, hardly the same family that arrived here last weekend. Do I have faith that these changes will be permanent? The skeptics say lasting change is unlikely. The scientists say prove it. Give us long-term follow-up data.

Maybe I'm afraid to find out that the improvements are only temporary. When kids who attend regular diabetes camp return to their homes, they stay motivated for a few months but then slowly slip back into their previous behaviors. I think I'm realistic. Of course, one week can't completely change old established habits and relationships. We aren't claiming that this week transforms all campers into happy, optimistic, sensitive family members. But we do know what their evaluations say at the time. I remember this one mother's words because they were so poignant. She wrote, "Before camp, I felt confused, alone, and had no confidence, and I was very much afraid. I'm not afraid anymore. I have hope again." Maybe that's temporary, but if these people leave here thinking they can begin again, and with confidence, that's proof enough for me.

Heather, who must have been packing in her bedroom, calls out, "You ready to go over?"

"Sure," I call back. I slip on my shoes. Walking to her room, I say, "I'll finish packing after the campers have gone."

"Well, I'm leaving right after breakfast. My dog's waiting for me." We walk over to the lodge. Darryl has pulled his car up to the front to load up. Several other campers are carrying their bags to their cars. It always looks like so much more stuff going than coming. Maybe it's because no one packs, they just throw all the dirty laundry, shells, clay models, banners, and soiled mud-hike shoes into the trunk. That doesn't leave as much room for the suitcases.

Little Lucy and Emily busily sort out their beach treasures, which have been airing on the railing. The buckets, filled with more shells, also are emptied and sorted. What a great morning activity for these small ones. My daughter used to insist we bring home shells from each beach walk. Now we have an extraordinary collection of fairly ordinary shells.

Pat rings the bell for final announcements. "Looks as though you're all getting packed up. Please try to look all around for your things. Remember your musical instruments, your cameras, your toothbrushes, your reading material. There are some coats hanging over in the French House that might belong to some of you. If you do leave anything behind, we'll try to mail it to you. If you haven't handed in your evaluation form, please do before you leave. I think most of you have exchanged addresses, but I'll try and send out a printed list to you, along with reprints of some of the articles you have requested."

Heather says, "Most of you wanted the recipe for the baked beans and the zero dressing. I'll send those along, too."

I add, "If you get any good snapshots, send us a copy and we'll put it in our camp album. I'll send you a copy of the family shot I want to take before you leave. So please don't drive off until we've taken your picture." I enjoy taking these last photos.

"Does anyone have any questions?" Pat asks.

"What do you want us to do with the sheets?" Lisa asks.

"If you'll just put them at the foot of the stairs, that would be great."

"Anything else?"

"Pat, who's going to sleep in my bed next week?" Tate wants to know.

"I'm not exactly sure, but a camp full of fifth and sixth graders will be here for the next two weeks." Tate's toothless grin appears. "Shall we all go to breakfast?" The kids run over, as the adults enjoy the stroll.

When I enter the dining hall, Cindy waves to me. She's saved me a seat. At the head of the table, I have Becky on my left and Cindy on my right. She has her hair pulled back in two pigtails. So has Becky. They both look bright.

"Dr. Mac, when are you coming down to Port Clyde? Let me know and I'll come see you off. Kev and me like to watch the 'Laura B' load up. All them artists going to Monhegan are sort of weird. Do you know any of them?"

"Not really, I pretty much stick to myself on the island. It's a great getaway for me, and I don't do any socializing."

"That sounds boring" Cindy says, with a smile.

"'Tain't really," I say. Becky laughs at my meager attempt at Maine talk.

"Could you pass the French toast, please?" Peter, four seats down, wants another piece. Here we serve French toast with apple sauce and cinnamon. We usually leave the maple syrup off, although there are some brands of low-calorie syrup. Heather says she'd rather promote apples and cinnamon. Most everyone is willing to go with it. I've tried cottage cheese, and that's good, too. Becky sends the plate down to Peter.

"So, Becky, what will you be doing for the rest of the summer?"

"Well, I'm going to a music day camp. My clarinet teacher thinks I can make junior high orchestra this fall, if I practice."

Cindy adds, "You did a good job last night, Beck."

"Thanks, so did you. I hope your mom let's you try out for the show now. She looked happy to see you do so well with my mom."

"Yeah, last night before bed, she told me I could. I hope I get a part." This girl has come alive.

"It sounds like you two have some fun summer activities. Drop me a line and let me know how it all works out." Many campers do keep in touch, but if they live far way, we may never hear from them again. Perhaps, at Christmas, Pat and I will send cards to all the old campers. Some of the young kids who were here ten years ago are probably in college or have jobs by now. And the older ones might even be married.

Pat stands over near the kitchen door. "I think we should give a big cheer for Laurie. Laurie, come on out." The campers clap. Eddy and Ginny, who have enjoyed Laurie's affable disposition, cheer and clap the loudest. Eventually, Laurie comes to the doorway and waves. She thanks everyone for being so helpful in the kitchen and tells them to return. Then she retreats to her parlor.

"Becky, we need to get going," Darryl stands by our table. "Your mother is packing up the last few things, and then we'll have to go. It's quite a drive to Great Barrington."

"Can't we stay just a little longer?" Becky asks. "I want to say good-bye to everyone."

"Honey, somebody has to be the first to leave, and I'll bet everyone will be leaving soon, too."

Heather walks over to our table. "Well, I'm going to be leaving now. I hope you all will be back some time. It's really been fun getting to know you." Those at the table say their farewells to Heather. I tell her to have a good time fishing. She and her husband, with their trusty dog, canoe the northern Maine lakes and fish for landlocked salmon. She says good-bye to the last table of campers, has a few brief words with Laurie, and heads for her Subaru.

"Well, Dad, I guess you're right. Everyone will be leaving soon." Becky gets up, clears her plate and glass, and comes back to the table. "You'll be coming over to the lodge to say good-bye?" She looks at Cindy and me.

"Yep, we'll be right over. I need to get a picture of you and your parents before you head out for the wild west." As Darryl and Becky go out the door, other campers start getting up too. Very soon, the camp will be empty.

Pat, Ginny, Eddy, and I quickly finish off the dishes. Laurie, in her quiet way, has already started them soaking. We all walk back to the lodge. Noticing a light green Saab parked out front, Ginny runs into the lodge to find her uncle, who has come to pick her up. I've know him for several years. We were committee members on the United Way Board and participate in many American Diabetes Association events. Ginny's so proud of him. He's a fine lawyer.

"Dr. MacCracken, have you seen my soccer ball?" Peter looks worried. "Abigail and I have looked everywhere."

"Last I remember, you and Jeff were dribbling it around the porch, just before the talent show. Have you checked in the treasure chest?" He runs off with renewed hope.

The Ohio contingent is the first to be completely packed. With my trusty camera, I snap a family photo and find it symbolic that Darryl is in the center with his arms around his wife and daughter. They say good-bye to the other campers. Nancy hugs Kevin and Lydia. Embracing Cindy, Nancy encourages her to keep singing.

Then she and Darryl turn to Pat and me. "We're going to miss you all. It's been the best vacation we've had in a long time," Darryl says. "We sure wish you all lived closer, but we'll see you again, for sure."

He hugs us both and climbs into the driver's seat. "All aboard!" The car engine roars.

Nancy hugs Pat and then me. She whispers, "Thank you, so much. You've given me a new daughter and new husband."

"Maybe a new outlook on life," I add.

"Yes, I think so." With moist eyes, she climbs into the car.

Becky and Cindy have been talking together. Actually, these two girls have very little in common. But that hasn't stopped them from becoming good friends. Each fulfilled a need in the other.

"Becky, we need to go. Hop in, please." As Becky opens the car door, she hesitates for just a moment. She reaches into the backseat and hands Cindy her tiny yellow Walkman portable cassette tape radio.

"Mom and I want you to have this. Keep singing."

Cindy's eyes light up. "Becky, don't you need it?"

"I've got my CD player. Please take it."

"Thank you so much."

"And don't forget to write me," Becky adds.

"I'll write you tomorrow."

Slowly, the car rolls forward. "Drive carefully," Pat remarks.

The group of us wave and call out our good-byes. Darryl toots his horn as they proceed down the driveway.

One family gone.

The other families complete their packing. Emily and Little Lucy divvy up their shells. A major project. Kicking his soccer ball, Peter rounds the corner of the porch.

"I found it, Dr. MacCracken. How did you know where it was?"

"I've been around here a lot of years, Peter, and soccer balls almost always end up in the treasure chest." He fires the ball at me. I trap and return it.

"Peter," Mark calls, "we're about ready to leave. Lucy, honey, you need to finish up now. We can always find more shells on our beach. Let Emily have those last few." Little Lucy obediently scoops the last several into Emily's bag. Emily grins, for she has no beach around her house.

Abigail and her mother come outside. The Bar Harbor family gathers for their photo; Peter, with his foot on his soccer ball, Lucy, with her bag of shells, and Abigail, with her honorary nurse's hat. We'll see this family again, as soon as clinic starts up this fall. But this week gave us a wonderful chance to get to know each one of them better. This family, so new with diabetes, is on the right track. The strong family bonds will help Peter all along the way.

"It's been great, Doc . . . and Pat, thanks for all those special awards. I don't think Abigail is ever going to take off that hat." Mark touches his daughter on the back.

"Oh, Daddy," Abigail replies. She's used to her father's joking.

Her mother says, "Thanks a lot. We'll see you in September. And I may be calling you for some fine tuning of Peter's dosage."

"You know how to reach us," Pat adds.

Mark turns to Sam, shakes his hand, and says a few private words. Sam pats Mark's shoulder and says, "We'll probably see you at the clinic."

"OK, guys, everyone in the car." The kids all jump in the back seat, and instantly hang out the window. As the car pulls away, they shout, "Bye, Eddy! Bye, Ginny! Bye, Lucy! See ya, Jeff and Kyle! Bye, Kevin! Their voices fade. Their arms keep waving until they're out of sight. What a great family.

Our numbers are dwindling. Brent, Marjorie, Tate, and Susan gather around and say good-bye. Susan, purple sunglasses on her head, comes over for a hug. We've had some special times together. I may never see Susan again, but I'll certainly never forget her. Her color has improved, and her face looks less puffy. She hasn't had any bad reactions for several days. Too much insulin can have such a devastating effect on kids.

I snap a shot of the Philadelphia family and then Brent takes one of Pat and me with our arms around the counselors.

"Well, I'll send you a copy, if it comes out." Most of Brent's photos do.

"Great," Pat replies.

Brent and his family climb in their car. They'll be staying in Maine for a few more days, I guess. Marjorie, eager to see her other two children, waves farewell. It won't surprise me if they settle in Blue Hill, someday.

"See you next year," Tate shouts. We all wave.

As their car pulls out, another pulls in. It's Eddy's family. Eddy jogs over to the car. His two little twin sisters pop out of the car, stretching their legs. It's a couple hours ride from Augusta. He hugs Marissa and Marie, who looks great. I haven't seen her for awhile, but diabetes hasn't seemed to slow her down. Pat walks over to say 'hi', and Marie gives her a big hug. As I watch Eddy's family gather around him, Pearl comes up behind me. She stands there a second and says, "He's a fine young man, that Eddy. Sam certainly enjoyed talking with him. You made a good choice in bringing him."

"You're right, Pearl. He's done a good job."

"I think I'll just go right over there and tell his parents so." She walks right over to the group. Eddy and Pat step aside and introduce Pearl. I see her shake hands with Eddy's parents and the twins. Immediately, she's giving them a piece of her gentle mind. As grandmother and mother, Pearl knows what compliments mean. And Eddy's parents have good reason to be proud.

Sam and Emily carry the last of their things to their truck. Walking back, Sam puts his daughter on his shoulders. Emily bounces up and down, holding on to her father's head. Pearl leaves Eddy and joins her family. They walk over to say good-bye.

"Thanks for everything," Pearl says.

"You were right, Doc. We're glad we stayed," Sam adds. "I promise we'll come down in a few months. And I'll get that eye appointment, too."

"That's good. Come visit us anytime. Now why don't you three stand over by this tree, and I'll take a picture." Sam puts one arm around his mom and holds Emily's feet with the other. Emily's hands cover Sam's forehead. All three grin.

Breathless, Jeff and Kyle appear from nowhere. If Sam's leaving, they must be here to say good-bye. Steve and Lucy are walking slowly up from the field. They must have gone down to show Steve the beach. Jeff asks if I'll take a picture of his family with Sam's. I agree, and Jeff yells for his mom and dad to hurry.

"There's no hurry, Jeff," Sam says. "We can wait."

Sam takes Emily down from his shoulders.

"Dr. MacCracken, I guess we're going to go now." Ginny stands nearby with her uncle.

I comment to Ginny's uncle about her successful week here, while Ginny says good-bye to everyone near me and then walks over to give a special farewell to Eddy and Pat. Her uncle hops into his car. She throws her last few belongings into the Saab. Then she walks over to Cindy, who has been quietly sitting off by herself. During this week, these two talked late into the nights. Cindy has made some meaningful connections. Saying good-bye is hard. The two talk for a few moments. Ginny gives Cindy a hug and goes back to the car. She waves to everyone as they pull out. Cindy waves, too.

Jeff taps my arm. "We're all here, Dr. MacCracken," He has arranged his parents in the back row with Sam, Pearl, and Emily. Kyle, and he are in the front. I snap a shot of seven smiling faces.

Steve shakes Sam's hand. "Thanks for taking care of my family while I was away."

"You got that wrong, Steve. They took care of me. You have a lovely wife and two great boys." Jeff and Kyle grab Sam's hands.

"Daddy, Mommy, can they come to our house for lunch. It's on the way to Houlton, isn't it?

"Sure, it's on the way. We live just north of Bangor, right off Route 95. We'd love to have you, if you'd come." Lucy smiles.

Sam looks at Pearl and Emily. Why not? They'll have to stop for lunch somewhere. Too far to make it all the way home. "Sure, that would be great." The kids cheer with excitement. They run to their vehicles.

Pearl, Sam, Lucy, and Steve say good-bye to the remaining group and take off. Near the end of the long driveway the car and truck stop.

Sam's probably asking directions to the lunch stop.

I turn around and see Cindy, Kevin, and Lydia, sitting on the porch bench. No one looks too eager to leave. For them, there is no hurry. Perhaps they are just enjoying the last few moments of spacious living. Their belongings, still piled in the corner, are in garbage bags. They have no suitcases. Cindy's new Walkman is attached to her belt, the earphones hanging around her neck. I hope those earphones don't break the line of communication that has just been reopened with her mom. Lots of teenagers use those things to tune out the world, their parents, and their problems.

Kevin looks content to stay forever. Here he does not have to face Lou, his mother's boyfriend. Here his mother's attention has been undivided. Perhaps he listened to Sam's story of how helpful his stepfather has been. Perhaps he knows his mother needs some adult companionship. Maybe he can see a better life ahead with another income in the family. For a boy of twelve, he has a lot to think about, to worry about. I'm afraid there are no miracles here for this family. They'll have no easy road. Small steps will require big efforts. Are they ready to try. I'm just not sure.

Eddy and his family come over to say good-bye. I recognize Eddy's mother but haven't seen his father for several years. Eddy looks just like his dad, only Eddy is about two inches taller and has no pot-belly. Mr. Jelkepski shakes my hand with his two. "It's nice to see you again. It's been a long time, seven years I think. Thanks for having my boy for a week. We missed him, but he says he had a good time."

"He was a great help to everyone here. I hope he'll consider helping us again next year." As the twins help their brother load up the car, Pat explains that Eddy is feeling better about Marie's diagnosis.

Eddy's father says, "So glad to hear that. He's been so worried about her. His mother and I, we know she'll be OK, just like our boy Eddy." It's a joy to see this family, so much love, admiration, and hope.

"Pop, we're all set." Eddy says good-bye to Kevin and his family. He looks over at me as he leaves them. I know he's wondering whether Kevin will thrive. I try to give him an optimistic glance.

"Well, thanks again for having me, Doc. Oh, and thanks again for those tickets. My dad and I will enjoy them. And those Red Sox better win, when we're there."

"You should be that lucky," says Kevin, who has walked up to the car.

"Hope to see you around Kev, maybe here next year?"

"Maybe." Kevin replies.

The car pulls away. Pat, Kevin, Cindy, and Lydia wave along with me. We're all going to miss Eddy.

Pat and I glance at each other. These good-byes have taken a little longer than we figured. By now, both of us are eager to get ourselves packed up and get home to our own families. We can't exactly kick the last family out, but from past experiences, we recall that some folks never want to go.

"Let me help you load up your car, Lydia." I'm not terribly tactful sometimes, but they appear to be in a state of inertia.

"I'll drive it around," she replies. She digs into her purse for the keys, and walks to her car. Kevin and Cindy help Pat and me move the pile out to the turnaround. When Lydia swings the car around, we start to load. With the back hatch open, the odor of old fish is evident. The back is full of small pieces of lobster shells, old soda cans, and used brown bags. A couple of orange syringe tops lie on the floor. Kevin and Cindy throw the garbage bags in. Lydia turns off the motor. The car obviously could use a new muffler, too.

She gets out. "This car better hold together for a few more years. She's rusting from all that sea salt, and the muffler damn near fell off last week. Lou strapped it back on with some wire. Don't know how long that'll last, though. He says . . ."

Kevin interrupts, "Mom, it'll hold. Lou knows cars." Kevin is oblivious to the significance of his positive statement.

Cindy smiles ever so slightly and winks at me. "We better get

237

going, Mom. I'm sure Pat and Dr. MacCracken want to leave, too."

I smile. "Well, we are looking forward to seeing our families. But we really enjoyed meeting you three. I hope you can come back next year. It would be fun to be together again. And I really want you to come to Bangor to see Dr. Rogers and stop in to see us. Our offices are pretty close."

"I'll try to come, but a lot depends on our transportation. As long as this car stays running, we'll be fine."

I'm not optimistic that they'll make it. But that doesn't mean we shouldn't keep encouraging them. "And thanks again for the lobster figures. Mine's going on my desk back at work. Come see it."

Pat gives each of them a hug. I do the same. Lydia and Kevin get in the front. Cindy gets in the back. She reaches her hand out to grab Pat. It's almost a grasp for hope. Her eyes reflect joy and sadness at the same time, if that's possible.

We wave until the car is out of sight. Then Pat and I walk slowly back to the porch. Emotionally exhausted, we sit for a moment on the steps. We did it. One more year of Camp Kee-to-Kin draws to a close. This was quite a year. But we say that every year. For weeks we'll recall events of camp—the talent show, the seizure, the miracle, the flowers. These campers will be just names to our families and friends back home. The experience will be too hard to describe. I know. I've tried.

Pat says, "So, are you ready to do this again?" She looks at me with a smile.

"Well, maybe next year." We both laugh.

While Pat finishes a few financial matters in the office, I stop off at the French House to say good-bye to Laurie. She's already preparing for the next campers, who arrive tomorrow. It amazes me how she can do this all summer. And such great food, too.

"Laurie, thanks for the week. And remember, any time you want to come to my house and whip up a few of those great casseroles for my freezer, just let me know!"

"I may just be coming up to Bangor this fall. I'll give you a call."

"Take care. Have a good summer."

"You too, and say hi to your family for me." We only came here once as a family, but Laurie has always remembered them.

I stroll back to my room to load my Subaru, which is in better running shape than Lydia's—but not much tidier. While resting my file box on my knee, I awkwardly open the back of my car and notice a small brown bag with a yellow sticky note attached. The handwritten note reads, "Dr. Mac—thanks for everything. This week has been terrific. You'll never know what an oasis this was for us at this time. We want you to have this. Hope to see you soon. All our love, Pearl, Sam, and Emily."

I put down the file box and reach into the brown bag. I pull out the bronze plaque that Pearl had on her dresser all week. How did she know. What a beautiful gift. I read its words slowly.

Prayer of St. Francis

Lord, make me an instrument of your Peace.
Where there is hatred, let me sow love.
Where there is injury, pardon.
Where there is doubt, faith.
Where there is despair, hope.
Where there is darkness, light.
Where there is sadness, joy . . .

My eyes well up with tears. It's been another good year.

Epilogue

At the end of July, we received a package from Brent. It contained a great photo of Pat, Heather, and me singing our farewell song and enlargements of three other favorite shots. His note mentioned they had changed physicians and were looking forward to working with Susan's new doctor.

Brent invited me to Philadelphia for a squash match—anytime. His wife wrote to thank Heather for the recipes and to let us know that Susan had lost a few pounds and looked great. She also said Tate was still talking about Camp, Eddy, and moving to Maine. She thanked us all for the week.

Sam, Emily, and Pearl come to clinic every three months. Sam is now assistant manager of his stepfather's building company, and Emily is thriving in kindergarten. They keep in touch with Jeff and his family, occasionally seeing each other at the clinic visits. Jeff's mom, Lucy, had hip surgery last month and is recovering slowly. But that hasn't stopped her from organizing the kids' diabetes support group.

We haven't heard anything from the Ohio family. I hope Nancy continues her singing and Darryl stays involved with Becky. Perhaps, she will do a science project on diabetes. We'll probably never know. Or then again, maybe Becky will someday apply for the counselor job at Camp, or maybe her folks will stop by on the way to that second honeymoon on Penobscot Bay.

Mark and Lisa moved from Bar Harbor to South Portland for better jobs. So far, they still come to our clinic, but after a few trips, I think they may find the two and a half hour drive too much. Peter looks great, enjoying his new fifth grade. We haven't seen Abigail (she doesn't want to miss school), but her little sister Lucy still comes with her mom or dad and Peter. She told me on their last visit that she wants to be an animal doctor. She said, "Cats get diabetes, too."

Of course, I'd like to tell you that Cindy starred in the musical and Lou and Lydia are married, living happily with Kevin and his sister. Dr. Rogers did see them for two sessions. But they've failed to keep their last three appointments. Maybe the old car fell apart. Kevin's social worker did call a few weeks ago, though, to tell me that, although she hasn't seen him recently, he hasn't been in the hospital since before camp. She wanted to know just what we had done to halt his hospitalizations. Then she quickly added, "Oh, by the way, I have another family that could use your help."

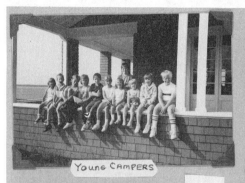
YOUNG CAMPERS

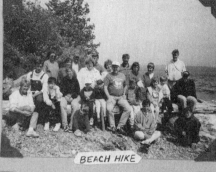
BEACH HIKE

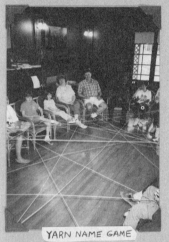
YARN NAME GAME

THRU THE YEARS

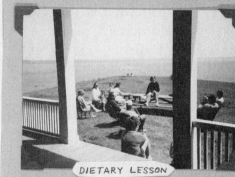
DIETARY LESSON

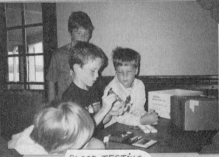
KIDS' INSTRUCTION

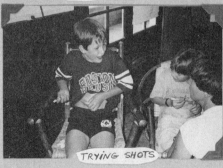
BLOOD TESTING

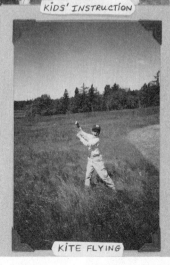
KITE FLYING

TRYING SHOTS

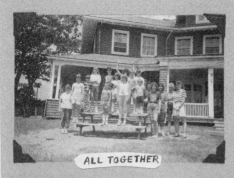
ALL TOGETHER

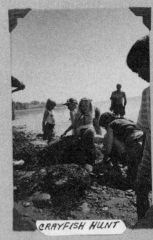
CRAYFISH HUNT

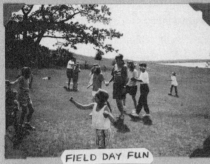
FIELD DAY FUN

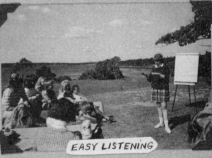
EASY LISTENING

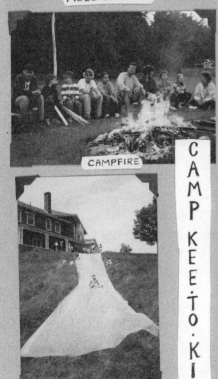
CAMPFIRE

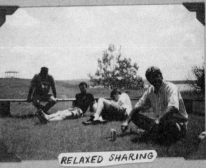
RELAXED SHARING

CAMP KEE·TO·KIN

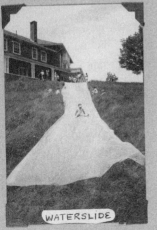
WATERSLIDE

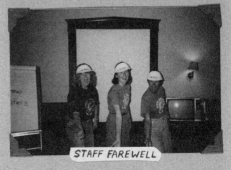
STAFF FAREWELL

Glossary

Autoimmune system—A system of specialized cells and messengers that can track what is foreign in the body. Antibodies (proteins) are produced by these specialized cells against foreign substances. But occasionally the immune system produces antibodies against "self," thus autoimmune, and attacks what is not foreign. Antibodies against the pancreas and its insulin-producing cells occur in diabetes.

Carbohydrate Counting—A newer method of meal-planning for people with diabetes based on total carbohydrates, paying less attention to complex carbohydrates (starches) and simple sugars allowing more flexibility in food choices within the carbohydrate groups. A fairly sophisticated approach attempting to match insulin dosage to total carbohydrate. Healthy choices still need to be encouraged.

Counterregulatory hormones—Those hormones within the body secreted by various endocrine glands during stress, which raise the blood glucose (sugar), thus having the opposite effect of insulin, which lowers blood glucose. These hormones include epinephrine (adrenaline), glucagon, cortisol, and growth hormone.

Dawn phenomenon—A rise in blood sugar in the early morning occurring before eating. It is thought in part to be due to the nighttime secretion of growth hormone and usually occurs more commonly in rapidly growing adolescence.

Glucagon—A hormone produced by the pancreas that raises blood glucose levels. With severe low blood sugar (an insulin reaction), glucagon can be injected to help raise the blood glucose level.

Glycosylated hemoglobin (hemoglobin A1c)—A blood test that indicates the average blood glucose level over the previous three months. The test is used to monitor diabetes control.

HLA system (complex)—A group of related genes located on Chronosome 6. These genes determine several proteins on the cell surface that are important in determining acceptance or rejection of tissue transplants and in maintaining the function of the immune system. Certain combinations of HLA genes have been associated with increased susceptibility to specific diseases.

Honeymoon period—That time after the diagnosis of diabetes when insulin doses are low and the person's pancreas still is producing some insulin. This is a time when control is relatively smooth and easy.

Hyperglycemia—High blood glucose (hyper=high, glyc=glucose, emia=in the blood).

Hypoglycemia—Low blood glucose (hypo=low, glyc=sugar, emia=in the blood).

Insulin—A hormone produced in the beta cells of the pancreas that helps the body use glucose. It causes the blood glucose level to fall and is the key to getting glucose into the cells so it can be used for energy. People with Type I diabetes do not produce enough insulin and must get it by injection.

Ketoacidosis— See Ketones below.

Ketones—Breakdown products of fat, which are acids. Ketones can be used as fuel when glucose is not available to the cell. They may be present when there is insufficient insulin or when there are many stress (counterregulatory) hormones. Ketones give the breath a fruity smell. Too many ketones can lead to a dangerous situation called diabetic ketoacidosis. Many children are admitted to the hospital at the time of diagnosis with diabetic ketoacidosis.

Lipohypertrophy—Lumps in the fatty areas where insulin injections have been given. These are caused by overuse of the same spot. Injecting into these areas may cause erratic absorption of insulin.

Macular edema—Swelling of the back of the eye at the macula (important area of vision). This can be caused by poor diabetes control. Treatment is available with laser therapy.

Neuroglycopenia—Low glucose in the brain, which will lead to symptoms of irritability, headache, confusion, sleepiness, and eventually seizures and coma.

NPH insulin—A type of insulin that has its effect several hours after injection. Usually called an intermediate-acting insulin, it peaks six to eight hours after injection but this varies with each person and with the type of NPH. In the bottle it has a cloudy appearance and sometimes is referred to as the "cloudy" insulin.

Pancreas—A gland located behind the stomach that produces hormones including insulin and glucagon. In Type I diabetes the pancreas is damaged and fails to produce enough insulin and sometimes glucagon.

Polydipsia—Excessive thirst

Polyuria—Excessive urination

Rebound—An abnormally high blood glucose seen after an episode of low blood glucose. It is thought to be caused by the body's emergency secretion of counterregulatory hormones.

Regular insulin—The type of insulin that acts fairly soon after injection and peaks in one to two hours. It is usually given before meals. It is clear in the bottle, compared with NPH, which is cloudy.

Somogyi phenomenon—Another name for rebound, named after the man who first described this observation of hyperglycemia after hypoglycemia (high sugar following low sugar).

Other Books on Diabetes

Raising a Child with Diabetes, Linda Siminerio, RN, MS, CDE, and Jean Betschart, RN, MN, CDE, American Diabetes Association, 1995.

The Take-Charge Guide to Type I Diabetes, American Diabetes Association, 1994.

Necessary Toughness: Facing Defenses and Diabetes, by Jonathan Hayes with Robert L. Briggs, American Diabetes Association, 1993.

Parenting a Diabetic Child: A Practical, Empathetic Guide to Help You and Your Child Live with Diabetes. Gloria Loring. Lowell House, Los Angeles 1991.

Grilled Cheese at Four O'Clock in the Morning by Judy Miller, American Diabetes Association, 1988.

Journey of a Diabetic, Larry Pray, Simon and Schuster, 1983.

Resource and Support Organizations

American Diabetes Association (ADA)
1600 Duke Street
Alexandria, VA 22314
1-800-232-3472

Juvenile Diabetes Foundation International
432 Park Avenue South
New York, New York 10016-8013
1-800-223-1138

American Association of Diabetes Educators
444 North Michigan Avenue, Suite 1240
Chicago, IL 60611
1-800-338-3633

International Diabetic Athletes Association
6829 North 12th Street, Suite 205
Phoenix, Arizona 85014
1-602-433-2113

Medic Alert Foundation
(for information on medical identification bracelets and necklaces)
PO Box 1009
Turlock, CA 95381-9009
1-800-432-5378

To order more copies of

The Sun, The Rain, and The Insulin

Growing Up With Diabetes

Please send your requests to:

Tiffin Press of Maine
P. O. Box 549
Orono, Maine 04473

Enclose payment payable to *TIFFIN PRESS OF MAINE.*

Cost: $12.95 per book, plus $2.55 shipping and handling.
  Maine resident please add 6% (75¢) sales tax.

Discounts available on orders of 10 or more copies.

Be sure to include your:

  Name
  Address
  City, State, Zip
  Phone Number